What makes this book particularly of interest is that the author is a conventional medicine provider, working in a large, comprehensive medical center, who has successfully integrated alternative modalities into his practice.

— Douglas Hanes, PhD, Associate Professor, School of Research and Graduate Studies; Chair, Master of Science in Integrative Medicine Research, National University of Natural Medicine

Clinicians interested in the topic, or discouraged by vexing problems in clinical practice (as Drs Elder have been) would also like to have the material in this book as part of their tool kit, as would clinicians trying to come up with an appropriate and helpful way to assist their patients in navigating all the different care systems available.

The most interested will be the consumer who wants to improve their health or self-management of chronic conditions and is open to an Ayurvedic approach. And there certainly is a need for clinician-focused books on this topic.

— Keith H. Bachman, MD, Internal Medicine, Northwest Permanente; Medical Director for the Kaiser Permanente Northwest Severe Obesity/Bariatric Surgery program; Lead Physician for Weight Management for Kaiser Permanente's Care Management Institute

The audience should be individuals and health care providers with interest in healthy life style and approaches to chronic pain, based on Ayurveda and other complementary and integrative medicine approaches.

It is palpable that the authors have worked with these recommendations with many patients, and this makes the reader feel confident to try out the approaches.

— Tido von Schoen-Angerer, MD, MPH, Research, Associate ARCIM Institute, Filderstadt, Germany, and an Attending Pediatrician, Fribourg Hospital, Switzerland

The techniques and approaches reviewed in this chapter are experiential. It is helpful to report more experiences with each treatment prescription, with case studies, to make those experiences more accessible, which the authors have done.

With increased interest among my Kaiser Permanente colleagues in plant-based diets, I think there would also be an increased interest in Ayurveda, which I think is the main strength of this book.

— Lonnie J. Lee, MD, L.Ac, Family Medicine, Integrative Medicine Specialist, Mid-Atlantic Permanente Medical Group

Dr. Elder has a unique vantage point among medical doctors. He is ensconced in the values and practices of a medical delivery organization committed to examining what it does then seeking adjustments to get it right for patients. At the same time, he is an ayurvedic medicine practitioner imbued with decades-long commitment, with his physician spouse and co-author, to what may be called an ayurvedic lifestyle. I first came to know of Dr. Elder's work when he published outcomes of an ayurvedic medicine intervention in the peer-reviewed literature. His whole-system research approach remains a beacon in the research community for those wishing to respect traditional medicine principles. In this book, one senses all of these rivers of interest at play. Gratefully, one mainly finds the presence of two physicians with good bedside manner—or, better said, "life-side manner"—guiding one to the potential for ayurvedic choices and tastes in one's own health and healing. This book will be a life-enhancing resource for many.

—John Weeks, The Integrator Blog News & Reports, Editor in Chief, Journal of Alternative and Complementary Medicine (Paradigm, Practice and Policy Advancing Integrative Health)

PICTURE OF HEALTH

Transform your self-care and health care through Ayurvedic and Integrative Medicine

PICTURE OF HEALTH

Transform your self-care and health care through Ayurvedic and Integrative Medicine

Charles R. Elder, MD, MPH, FACP, & Leslie D. Elder, MD

Illustrated by Leslie D. Elder, MD

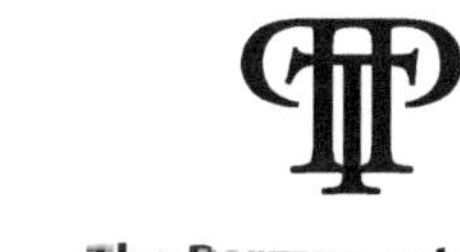

The Permanente Press
Portland, Oregon • Oakland, California

Published 2019 by The Permanente Press
Portland, Oregon • Oakland, California

The Permanente Press is owned by The Permanente Federation, LLC
Oakland, California

PICTURE OF HEALTH: TRANSFORM YOUR SELF-CARE AND HEALTH CARE
THROUGH AYURVEDIC AND INTEGRATIVE MEDICINE

23 22 21 20 19 1 2 3 4 5

ISBN: 978-0-9770463-8-6
Library of Congress Control Number: 2019944271

Artwork by Leslie D. Elder, MD
Book design by Lynette Leisure
Printed in the United States of America

For our sons,

Jacob Matthew and Isaiah James

TABLE OF CONTENTS

INTRODUCTION

A FEW THINGS THEY NEGLECTED TO MENTION IN MEDICAL SCHOOL

How did two primary care physicians become interested in complementary and integrative medicine, and how do we use it in our practice?

I, Charles Elder, was one of those guys who was born with stethoscope already in hand. Ancestors and fate apparently had preselected my career track in medicine quite some time before I was even conceived. After a 17-year incubation period in Northeast Ohio, and having finally completed high school, I grabbed my stuff, hopped into the family Buick, and headed East.

The next day, my dad dropped me off at Warren Towers at Boston University. This enormous dormitory housed 1800 students, 600 apiece in each of 3 adjacent towers. The location was excellent, with convenient access both to university resources and to all of Boston's amenities. However, with the Massachusetts Turnpike on the one side, and Storrow Drive, a major crosstown parkway, on the other, it presented, compared with my small hometown in Ohio, an intensely urban environment. On top of that, although at my Ohio high school I was a star student, the academic atmosphere in college was extremely competitive, and in my medical studies program at Boston University, I was just one of the pack. Needless to say, I felt highly stressed and wondered to myself, "Am I in over my head?"

Desperate for a creative solution, I sought out training in a wide variety of mind-body and stress management techniques. I visited the Zen Center, the Kundalini Yoga Center, and the Transcendental Meditation Center. I enrolled in a Tai Chi class at the University. I studied, or experimented with, a large number of other more obscure approaches and techniques as well. Many of these techniques I found to be compelling and beneficial. For me, the one most beneficial, and the one that stuck with me, was Transcendental Meditation. I found that if I had a tension headache, I would meditate, and the headache would go away! After hours of studying, I'd get brain fog and couldn't concentrate. Then I would meditate, clearing the cobwebs from my head, and I could again concentrate on my studies. "My gosh," I thought to myself, "this is *really* benefiting me."

I have continued to meditate on a regular basis since, and as relates to medical education, would offer two comments: 1) I surely would not have survived the rigors of medical training without this valuable stress reduction tool and 2) the experience of regular meditation practice radically shifted my perspective on medical training. Although I was very fortunate to receive an excellent education in biomedicine, I retained a nagging awareness that the model of care I was learning was fundamentally incomplete. We commonly managed patients with chronic dosing of potentially dangerous and addictive drugs, offering no attempt at or even mention of self-care approaches that I knew from personal experience to be extremely effective. "This patient has been into our emergency room 3 times during the past 2 weeks for demerol injections for his headaches. Why isn't anyone advising him to learn to meditate?" I would wonder. "This patient is taking 15 mg of valium daily to manage her anxiety, why isn't anyone telling her to meditate?" I found all this especially perplexing because I had been taught to value scientific evidence as a basis for therapeutics, and at that time there was already data in the literature supporting the use of mind-body approaches for such conditions.[1] When I was a student, the fact that safe, noninvasive, effective approaches were available but going unmentioned in favor of potentially hazardous drug therapy impressed me as strange. Today, having accrued 3 decades of clinical experience, it *still* impresses me as strange!

After graduating from medical school, I began my internship and residency training in internal medicine at the University of Michigan Hospitals in Ann Arbor, where I met my wife (LE), who was a resident physician in the family medicine program. Toward the end of our residency training, my wife said to me, "Hey, Charles, the Cleveland Transcendental Meditation Center is sponsoring a weekend meditation retreat at Oberlin next month. We should go." We attended the retreat and found it relaxing and enjoyable.

As it turned out, one of the speakers at the retreat was a prominent physician from the faculty at The Ohio State University School of Medicine, who gave an engaging talk about the research program in his laboratory investigating the antioxidant and antineoplastic properties of some traditional ayurvedic herbal formulas.[2,3] I found the talk fascinating. This was the first time I had heard about ayurveda, the traditional health care system of India. The experience inspired my wife and me to seek additional clinical training in ayurveda to supplement our conventional medicine skills. During the following years, through continuing education and fellowship training, we gained invaluable knowledge and skills in areas in which our conventional medicine training had been sadly lacking: diet, daily routine, exercise, mind-body medicine, herbal supplements, and the like.

After completing residency, we moved to Portland, Oregon, where I joined the medical staff at Kaiser Permanente Northwest. This has been a terrific place to practice, and I have had the privilege of serving as primary care physician to many thousands of Kaiser Permanente patients during a span of more than 25 years. But there is more to that story. After 5 or so years of full-time clinical work, I grew exceedingly frustrated with conventional primary care internal medicine practice. Burnout was setting in. In retrospect, I attribute this not to the work hours, but rather to the mismatch between the tools in my conventional medicine toolkit and the types of problems my patients actually presented with. Conventional medicine can be compelling and effective for the acutely ill patient, but for those with more chronic conditions, the paradigm often falls short. In addition, a substantial percentage of patients present to primary care medicine clinics not with a solitary crisp and clear concern, but rather with multiple complaints of a more vague or uncertain nature, and/or unrecognizable patterns of symptoms to which no diagnosis can be confidently assigned. (This is another important fact about medical practice that is not mentioned in medical school!) After about 5 years I finally had to ask myself, "Why are these patients coming to see me?" On many days, patients with chronic problems, such as musculoskeletal pain, depression, fatigue, irritable bowel, or fibromyalgia, represented the lion's share of the work, and yet these syndromes remain poorly understood, and are often inadequately managed, using a narrow, conventional medicine toolkit. At the same time, I had gained skills in a different paradigm, ayurveda, which I knew from my training, personal health practice, and the literature, to be potentially effective for such cases. Yet the conventional medicine system viewed the ayurvedic paradigm, and the types of holistic interventions it offers, as unorthodox. If, out of the blue, I started using them, I might land myself in trouble.

Eventually I submitted a written proposal to my supervisors. First, I pointed out that many patients presenting to primary care internists bring problems that are not always well managed using the prescription drugs we offer. This fact is obvious enough to most anyone spending significant clinical time in an outpatient internal medicine practice. I then described the ayurvedic approach to a number of these conditions, the prescribed interventions along with their rationale, and suggested a pilot program introducing this approach into my primary care practice. For specific subsets of patients, when clinically appropriate and with the patient's consent, we would attempt an ayurvedic dietary, behavioral, and herbal protocol. I developed a questionnaire instrument to be sent to patients a month after the consultation to find out if they were satisfied with their care, and if their condition had improved. During the period of a couple of months, I gathered data on about a dozen patients, with rave reviews.

These data favorably impressed my leadership team. The pilot project morphed into a referral-based clinic, where I provided integrative medicine consultations, coordinating ayurvedic prescriptions with conventional medical therapeutics, to a wider group of patients. Initially, I staffed this integrative medicine clinic one half-day a month, then a half-day a week, and over time the clinic has grown to encompass a substantial percentage of my practice. I am grateful to Kaiser Permanente Northwest for providing the opportunity to develop this program, which has been essential for both the welfare of many of our patients as well as my own professional satisfaction.

There remained, however, a significant logistic hurdle. Ayurveda is radically different from conventional medicine. The concepts, approach, and paradigm are foreign to the community we serve. How can a physician, during the course of a typical 20-minute office visit, orient the patient to understand the rationale and approach underlying a multimodality ayurvedic prescription? To solve this dilemma we introduced a unique program featuring group clinics. At our integrative medicine clinic, the patient's first appointment is not an ordinary visit with the physician, but rather a 2-hour group visit, attended by the physician (CE) along with typically 6 to 10 patients. At this group appointment, patients learn the fundamental vocabulary and paradigm of ayurveda, and receive a set of general dietary and lifestyle recommendations. Each patient returns home and begins implementing the self-care instructions. Then, a few weeks later, the patient returns for an individual consultation with the physician, at which time a full assessment takes place, and the physician prescribes an individually tailored treatment program.

Drawing upon our experience with thousands of patients, we developed this book to provide both a manual for patients seeking complementary and integrative care, and a source book for their physicians. The material in Chapters One through Six reviews and expands the curriculum from the introductory group visit, with the remaining chapters providing information, resources, and protocols to support each patient's individualized therapeutic program. Although many publications are available on both integrative medicine and ayurveda, this book offers timely contributions. The narrative reflects more than 2 decades of clinical experience practicing integrative medicine and ayurveda in a conventional managed care setting. How can health care organizations best integrate ayurveda, acupuncture, and other compelling approaches in ways that are authentic, feasible, useful to both patients and physicians, compatible with the conventional medicine culture, and scalable? This book provides new direction. We aim to empower both patients and physicians to evolve beyond the prevailing confusion in the complementary and integrative medicine arena. We believe you will find inspiration, clarity, insights, and ideas that will enable you to relieve symptoms, reverse health challenges, and optimize wellness.

Finally, although the text reflects our integrative medicine practice in Oregon, we created much of the content, including most of the artwork (by Leslie Elder), in 2017 while on sabbatical in Jerusalem. We wish to express our gratitude to Northwest Permanente for sponsoring the sabbatical, and for making this project possible.

— Drs. Charles & Leslie Elder

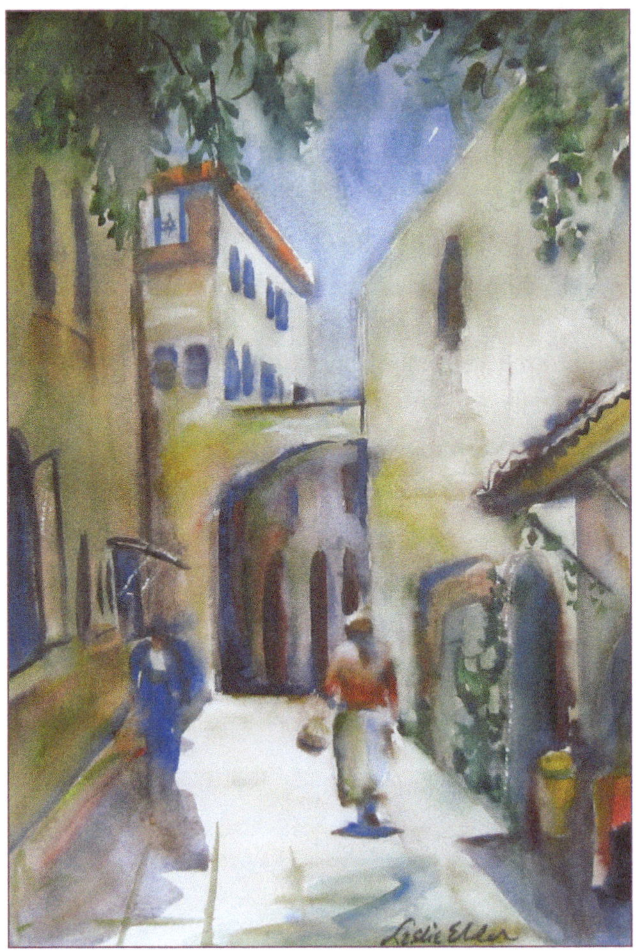

Woman in the Old City

(watercolor)

People of diverse religions and beliefs come to Jerusalem to draw closer to the source of all holiness. Ayurveda, likewise, is for everyone, providing systematic, time-tested guidelines for advancing people of all backgrounds toward ideal health.

PART I: THE BASICS

The basics of self-care
everyone needs to know

CHAPTER ONE

A BRAND NEW OLD IDEA

Ayurveda, an ancient system of holistic health care, provides fresh insights into how to maintain and improve your health.

When exploring systems of complementary medicine, in contrast to conventional medicine, one finds a different paradigm for evaluating the patient. In conventional medicine, we generally default to a "billiard ball" approach to analyzing disease causation: This germ causes that infection, this strained muscle causes that pain syndrome, and so forth. The thinking is linear. In the complementary medicine systems, in contrast, practitioners think more in terms of balance and imbalance. Health is a state of balance, or harmony, whereas disease is a state of imbalance, or having somehow gotten out of sync, or out of whack. From a clinical standpoint, then, complementary medicine practitioners tend more toward a systems approach to thinking about disease and health.

If health is a state of balance and disease a state of imbalance, the next logical question for consideration must be balance or imbalance of what? We will address this question from the vantage point of a system called *ayurveda*, which is the traditional health care system of India. Ayurveda is to India as Chinese medicine is to China, and is useful for us to consider for several reasons. First, ayurveda has been continuously practiced for thousands of years and is likely the oldest continuously practiced system of holistic care in the world. Indeed, scholars generally date the *Caraka Samhita*,[4] a fundamental textbook of ayurveda, to approximately 500 BCE, with the oral tradition being even older. Practically speaking, this indicates that most of the other complementary medicine paradigms currently prevalent and popular, such as Chinese medicine and naturopathy, will share a lot with, or will have borrowed a lot from, ayurveda. Second, scientists have published a considerable volume of research on ayurveda, especially in recent decades.[5,6] Most of this research has focused on mind-body techniques, yoga, and herbal mixtures, and, to a lesser extent, combined modality approaches.[7]

We can translate "ayurveda" as "knowledge of lifespan," and immediately we sense an approach quite different from what we are accustomed to. Of course ayurveda, as a health care system, offers a range of modalities for treating illness, including diet, herbals, exercise, yoga, mind-body techniques, daily routine, and more. The paradigm, however, fundamentally emphasizes prevention. To maximize healthy longevity, what foods do we eat, what routine do we follow, and what supplements do we take? According to the classic ayurvedic texts, the expected human lifespan is 120 years! Although this sounds ambitious, let's suppose you hope to live to the age of 100 years, while maintaining, for the most part, excellent health. With this goal in mind, what should you eat? All will agree that you wouldn't want the typical American diet, but exactly what type of diet should you follow? There's the raw-food diet, the gluten-free diet, the vegan diet, the Atkins diet, the South Beach Diet, the low-carb diet, the no-fat diet, the low-protein diet, the blood-type diet, the Paleo diet, and so on, seemingly ad infinitum. Little wonder people are confused. According to the oldest system of holistic health care in the world, what dietary patterns best support health and longevity over the span of a lifetime? Not this fad for 5 years, then on to the next fad for 3 to 4 years, then back to the previous fad. What diet best supports longevity and health, across the span of a lifetime, decade after decade? What is the daily routine and what are the exercise patterns that most effectively support health and longevity over the long haul? If you would like to know, then read on.

According to ayurveda, health is a state of balance, and disease a state of imbalance, of 3 fundamental physiologic, or "psychometabolic principles," called "doshas." The 3 doshas are called "vata," "pitta," and "kapha."

> **He whose doshas are in balance, whose appetite is good, whose dhatus are functioning normally, whose malas are in balance, and whose Self, mind, and senses remain full of bliss, is called a healthy person.**
> — Sushruta Saṃhitâ 15.41

What do these doshas mean? The first dosha, vata, governs all movement—mind, body, and spirit: movement of thoughts through the mind, movement of food through the digestive tract, movement of blood through the blood stream. Anything moving is under the domain of vata dosha. Pitta governs digestion, metabolism, and transformation. The whole process of eating something, then transforming what you have eaten into nutrients, is governed by pitta dosha. Kapha governs structure, the physical structure of the body. Tissues, organs, etc., the material body, fall under the domain of kapha dosha.

According to ayurveda, then, health is considered a state of balance and disease a state of imbalance of these 3 doshas: vata, pitta, and kapha. When the 3 doshas are balanced, i.e., present in the right amounts and functioning harmoniously together, 2 thumbs up! We're in good health. On the other hand, if one or more doshas becomes imbalanced, or overactive, because of improper diet, improper daily routine, some stress, some germ, some environmental toxin, or whatever other cause, this may tip the system out of kilter, with symptoms of illness potentially setting in. This, of course, represents a much different way of thinking about being healthy or not compared with what we are accustomed to encountering at the internal medicine or family medicine clinic.

Having said this, we will momentarily turn to a seemingly unrelated subject with the observation that different people have different natures, or constitutions. That is to say, some people are big, while others are little. Some people are quick, others slow. Some people remember things forever; others forget right away. Different people have different natures. The reason for introducing this point now is that in the ayurvedic system, we use the 3 doshas as a basis for classifying, or categorizing, people. In other words, some of us are vata types, some pitta types, some kapha types, and some various combinations. Although all of us have all 3 doshas governing our physiology, most of us, by virtue of how we were born and have developed, are naturally inclined to express the qualities of 1 or 2 doshas more than another. We will thus use these doshas to assign each patient a constitutional type: vata, pitta, kapha, or some combination thereof. Knowing one's ayurvedic body type provides guidance as to how one should best manage his/her health. After all, in the face of a given set of health concerns, what's right for one person might be wrong for the next, depending upon who that person is and how s/he is built.

Next, we will do as an exercise a body-type questionnaire (see figure on next page). The questionnaire serves as a tool to help familiarize ourselves with these concepts of vata, pitta, and kapha. The first part of the questionnaire is the vata part, the second part is the pitta part, and the third part is the kapha part. In the first part, the first item reads "I tend to do things quickly." If you are extremely quick, circle 5; if you tend somewhat toward being quick, circle 4; if you are exactly in the middle, circle 3; if you tend somewhat toward being slow, circle 2; if you are extremely slow, circle 1. Continue on down the page with responses to all 12 items. Specifically, answer the questions describing how you have been most of the time during the past year or so. After you have completed all the items for the vata part, total your score and write the total in the bottom right box. This is your score for vata dosha. Next, do the same in part 2 for pitta, and again the same in part 3 for kapha. When you are done, you will have tabulated a personal score for each of the three doshas.

Vata section	1. Does not apply at all	2.	3. Applies somewhat	4.	5. Applies a great deal
I tend to do things quickly.	1	2	3	4	5
I become anxious easily.	1	2	3	4	5
I learn quickly.	1	2	3	4	5
I forget things easily.	1	2	3	4	5
I have a thin physique.	1	2	3	4	5
I have a tendency toward constipation.	1	2	3	4	5
I am intolerant of cold, windy weather.	1	2	3	4	5
I tend toward dryness of the skin.	1	2	3	4	5
My sleep tends to be interrupted.	1	2	3	4	5
I am talkative.	1	2	3	4	5
I have difficulty making decisions.	1	2	3	4	5
I have a difficult time gaining weight.	1	2	3	4	5
				Total score:	

Pitta section	1. Does not apply at all	2.	3. Applies somewhat	4.	5. Applies a great deal
I am very focused and efficient in my work.	1	2	3	4	5
I get angry very easily.	1	2	3	4	5
I do not like hot weather.	1	2	3	4	5
I have a tendency toward skin problems.	1	2	3	4	5
I become very uncomfortable if I miss a meal.	1	2	3	4	5
My stools tend to be loose.	1	2	3	4	5
I have a large appetite.	1	2	3	4	5
I have a tendency toward getting heart burn.	1	2	3	4	5
I perspire a lot.	1	2	3	4	5
My intellect is sharp.	1	2	3	4	5
I crave cold foods and drinks.	1	2	3	4	5
People think I have an intense personality.	1	2	3	4	5
				Total score:	

Kapha section	1. Does not apply at all	2.	3. Applies somewhat	4.	5. Applies a great deal
I work in a steady and methodical way.	1	2	3	4	5
I do not have a big appetite.	1	2	3	4	5
It takes me a long time to learn new things.	1	2	3	4	5
I remember things a long time.	1	2	3	4	5
I have a large physique.	1	2	3	4	5
I do not like cold damp weather.	1	2	3	4	5
I tend not to perspire very much.	1	2	3	4	5
I tend to get lethargic.	1	2	3	4	5
My skin is oily.	1	2	3	4	5
I easily gain weight.	1	2	3	4	5
I sleep very soundly.	1	2	3	4	5
My bowel movements are regular.	1	2	3	4	5
				Total score:	

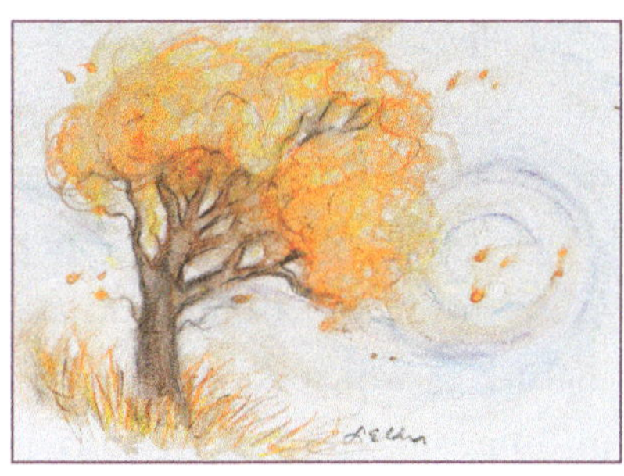

Before reviewing the interpretation of these questionnaire scores, let's learn more about the 3 doshas.

The first dosha, vata, governs all movement: mind, body, and spirit. Vata dosha, by definition, has these qualities: it is cold, moving, quick, dry, rough, light, and airy. Vata is composed of the elements space and air (see 3 doshas graphic below). People often liken vata to a snake. Not in the sense that snakes are a little creepy, if you think that, but rather in the sense that snakes demonstrate all of these qualities. The next time you see a snake in your garden, if you try to catch it, you will find it is not so easy. Snakes are quick, and they move. If you do manage to catch the snake and you pick it up, you'll find that is it is cold and light, and that its scales are rough and dry. Someone with a lot of vata in his or her physiology, when balanced, naturally expresses the following qualities: quick and alert, light and energetic, excellent imagination, vitality, and immunity. Too much vata, or vata out of balance, can give rise to: anxiety,

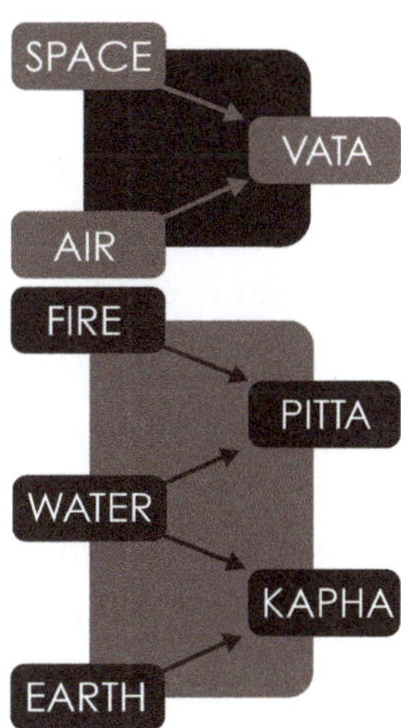

insomnia, constipation, high blood pressure, heart palpitations, excessive worry, dryness, and a range of similar medical problems and concerns.

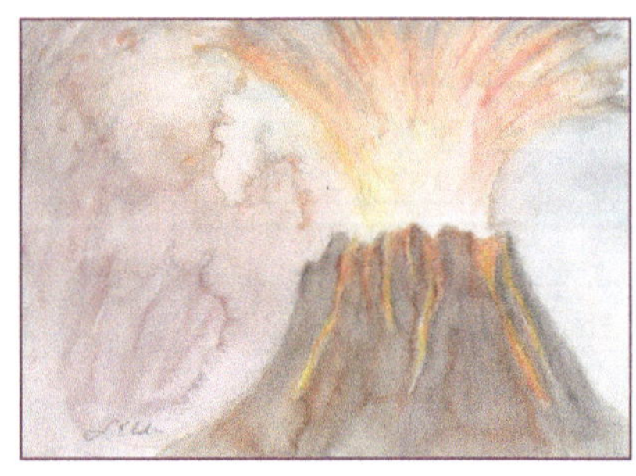

The second dosha, pitta, governs heat, digestion, metabolism, and transformation in the physiology. Pitta dosha encompasses the process of digesting one's food, and of transforming what we have eaten into nutrients. Pitta has these qualities: it is hot, sharp, moist, sour, and intense. Pitta is composed of the elements fire and water, and is often likened to the sun. When we think of pitta dosha, we think of the blazing hot sun on a July afternoon. Someone with a lot of pitta in his or her physiology, when balanced, naturally expresses these qualities: dynamic, efficient and productive, excellent leader and public speaker, and a sharp intellect. Too much pitta, or pitta out of balance, gives rise to heartburn, anger, temper flares, and skin rashes. Any inflammatory condition involves at least in some measure imbalance of pitta dosha.

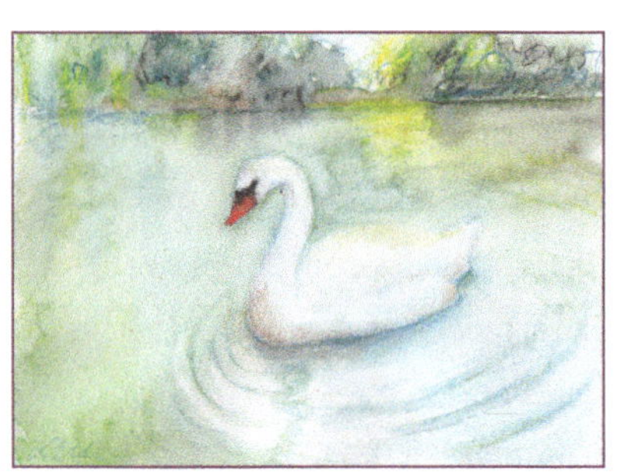

The third dosha, kapha, governs structure and lubrication of the mind, body, and spirit. Kapha dosha is heavy, sweet, steady, soft, and slow. Kapha is composed of the elements water and earth, and the animal in nature to which Kapha is often likened is a swan. Someone with a lot of kapha in his or her physiology, when balanced, naturally expresses these qualities: tranquil, steady, generous, firmly built, and affectionate. Too much kapha, or kapha out of balance, gives rise to depression, weight gain, obesity, diabetes, excess mucus production, sinus and respiratory conditions, and a range of similar medical problems or concerns.

Let's now turn back to consideration of the questionnaire scores. The questionnaire serves as an educational tool, and there are no right or wrong answers. It is not a cause for concern if your scores are all high, or all low, or wherever they fall. The most interesting thing for you will be how these 3 scores compare with one another for you. As one example, consider someone having the following scores: vata 52, pitta 28, kapha 23. In this case, the patient scores much higher on vata, suggesting a vata constitutional type. As a second example: pitta 58, vata 53, kapha 30. In this case the pitta score is highest, with vata a close second, suggesting a pitta-vata constitutional type. All told, then, there are 10 possible combinations, or 10 ayurvedic constitutional types: One can be a vata type, a pitta type, or a kapha type; or vata-pitta, pitta-vata, etc. (see Figure: Ten Ayurvedic Constitutional Types).

Ten Ayurvedic Constitutional Types		
Vata	Pitta	Kapha
Vata-Pitta	Vata-Kapha	Pitta-Vata
Pitta-Kapha	Kapha-Pitta	Kapha-Vata
Vata-Pitta-Kapha		

In our first example, the patient scores by far the highest on vata, suggesting a vata constitutional type. Many patients show what we can call a "monodoshic" pattern. Such people strongly demonstrate qualities of one particular dosha, as this example suggests. This is very important information to know about the patient. Vata types are most prone to vata disorders. Reflecting back upon what we previously reviewed about the 3 doshas, we recall that knowing one's constitutional type provides a window into the patient's strengths and vulnerabilities. Even if the patient is perfectly healthy, we can provide the individual with dietary, herbal, lifestyle, and other recommendations, all with a focus on reducing the influence of, or balancing, vata dosha.

In the second example, the pitta score is highest, with vata a close second, suggesting a pitta-vata constitutional type. Many people are "bidoshic," as this example suggests. In this sort of scenario, the prescription we provide for the patient might be seasonal. In the summer, when it's hot out, the patient needs to focus on balancing pitta dosha, while in the winter, when its cold out, the patient needs to focus on balancing vata dosha. If you take someone who is a hot-head by nature, and you place him/her in the hot sun, how does that tend to go? Not so well, of course. This helps elucidate the general approach we take. If someone has a lot of pitta in his or her constitution, i.e., the patient has a lot of heat just by nature, then to keep that person out of trouble we need to cool him/her off. The last thing such a person needs is more heat.

How close do the top 2 dosha scores on the questionnaire need to be to establish a bidoshic, as opposed to monodoschic, body type? This is not set in stone. However as a general rule, we will tell patients that if the score for a particular dosha represents at least 30% of the total of the 3 scores added together, that dosha can be considered as part of the prakriti (body type).[8]

What if all 3 scores on the questionnaire are very close, or are even the same? Some people are tridoshic, but this is unusual. Sometimes the questionnaire scores are misleading or inaccurate. Some people will take a questionnaire like this, and their scores provide insight and clarity as to what is going on with them. Others complete the questionnaire and the results are unclear or puzzling.

What is the most common cause of confusion when completing a body-type questionnaire? Consider the following 2 concepts. Each person has a body type, called the *prakriti*, as well as, potentially, any imbalance, called the *vikriti*. As previously suggested, the body type predicts the imbalance, that is to say, the prakriti predicts the vikriti. Vata types are most prone to vata imbalances, whereas pitta types are most prone to pitta imbalances, and kapha types are most to kapha imbalances. In this way, knowing one's body type provides the patient insight as to potential health-related vulnerabilities. However, this simple scenario doesn't always play out. In the real world, sometimes a pitta type can develop a kapha imbalance, or a vata type may develop a pitta imbalance, and so on. An imbalance in some other dosha that has developed can skew the scores on a body-type questionnaire, rendering the instrument more difficult to interpret.

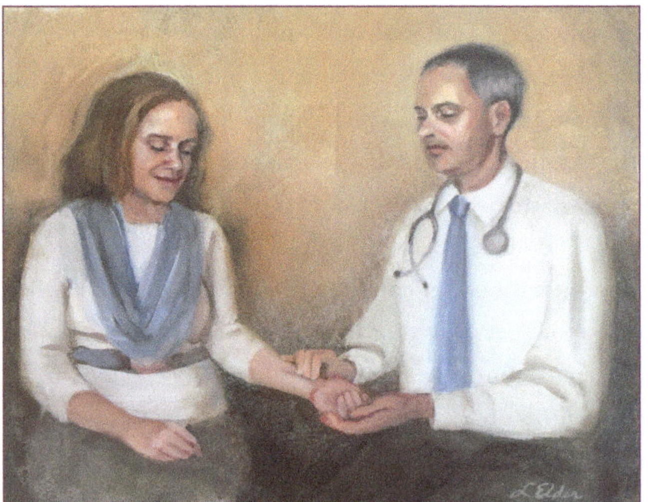

Taking the Pulse

(oil on canvas)

The physician performs ayurvedic pulse diagnosis. Through this technique, the physician discerns the relative balance of the doshas (vata, pitta, and kapha) and can identify blockages and impurities in the system. This process provides diagnostic and therapeutic insight of particular value in cases where conventional medicine approaches fall short.

To sort this out, the patient may need to see an ayurvedic practitioner, with a full assessment including a clinical history and a physical examination. In ayurvedic diagnostics, one of the key procedures we use is a technique called pulse diagnosis. When you come to the internal medicine or family medicine clinic, and the physician takes your pulse, s/he assesses how fast the pulse is going and whether the pulse is regular or irregular. When performing an ayurvedic pulse assessment, the analysis of the pulse is considerably more sophisticated. The physician takes the pulse with three fingers, with each of these (index, middle, and ring finger) evaluating a different dosha (vata, pitta, and kapha respectively). The physician places the 3 fingers on the radial pulse just above the wrist, and applies a systematic protocol for analyzing what the radial pulse is doing that informs the determination of the body type, the imbalances, and other clinical parameters.

Ayurveda describes a seasonal cycle of the doshas, with summer as pitta season, winter as vata season, and spring as kapha season. We are all a little more pitta in the summer, a little more vata in the winter, and a little more kapha in the spring. There is likewise a lifetime cycle of the doshas. The first part of life, up to age 20 or so, represents the kapha period of life. The middle part of life, say from ages 20-60, represents the pitta season of life, whereas the last part of life, from around age 60 onward, represents the vata season of life. We are all a little more kapha when we are kids, a little more pitta in midlife, and a little more vata as we grow older. This means that the diseases of childhood tend to be kapha imbalances, whereas the diseases of aging tend to be vata imbalances. If you take your child or grandchild to the doctor, most of the time, what is it for? Usually a cold, ear ache, stuffy nose, asthma flare, or some type of respiratory congestion triggers the visit. We commonly bring kids to the doctor for excess mucus in the respiratory tract, which is a manifestation of excess kapha.

At the other end of the spectrum, the diseases generally associated with aging tend to be vata imbalances. For example, in the case of dementia, the mind has lost its grounding. In the case of osteoporosis, the bones are too brittle and light. Both stem from imbalance of vata dosha. Menopause represents the transition from the pitta to the vata season of life. When patients present with complaints of menopausal symptoms, we usually do not recommend the prescription of hormone supplements of any type (see Chapter Fifteen). Rather, we advise a program for balancing vata dosha, including the appropriate dietary prescriptions, behavioral changes, mind-body approaches, and herbal supplements.

We have now devoted considerable attention to summarizing a new, or actually very old, approach to thinking about our health. Well, so what? How does this help us?

Let's now delve into answering that question in a very pragmatic way. In the coming chapters, we will use this paradigm, or lens, as a tool to help us understand when and what we should eat, how we should exercise, what our daily routine should encompass, when we should use herbal supplements, and more.

CHAPTER TWO

WHEN DO WE EAT?

When and how to eat to optimize digestion and health.

According to ayurveda, good health and good digestion are essentially synonymous. In the ayurvedic system, we thus place strong emphasis on maintaining proper digestion. Why would we make a statement like this? Why such a strong emphasis on maintaining proper digestion? The figure shows a simple diagram to illustrate the point.

We eat a meal and digest it. When we digest the meal, we either do a good job or a bad job digesting the food. If we do a good job digesting the meal, we generate nutrients. If we do a bad job, toxins are produced. So it is really quite simple. We can again indicate names for these concepts. We'll call digestion "agni," which means fire; the nutritious product we'll call "ojas," and the toxic byproduct of poor digestion we'll call "ama." Interestingly, the Sanskrit term for digestion, "agni," is the root of the English word "ignite." When we think about our digestion, we should hold the image of something like a gas stovetop, or a campfire.

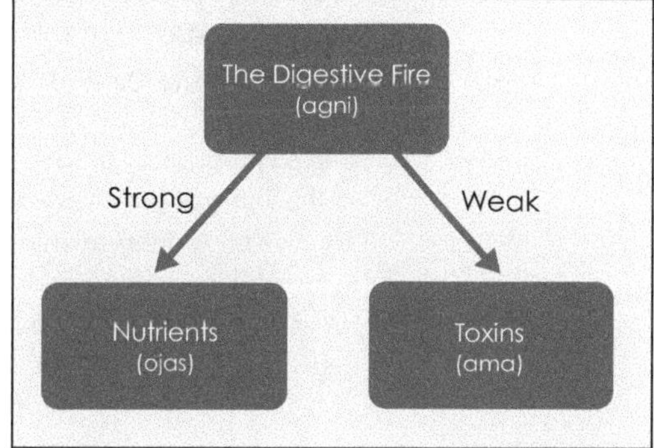

The Digestive Fire

We eat a meal, and if we are eating the right food at the right time, our digestion is strong, and everything is going our way; the product of a properly digested meal is a sweet, light, nutritious substance called ojas, which nourishes all the tissues of the body. However, what happens when we eat a meal, and we do a lousy job digesting the meal because digestion is weak, we are eating on the run, the food is unwholesome, or for whatever reason? The byproduct of an improperly or incompletely digested meal is a heavy, sticky, toxic substance called "ama." (see Sidebar: What Is Ama?) If the ama starts to accumulate in the physiology in any appreciable degree, it begins to deposit in the various tissues and organs of the body. Then, if some imbalanced dosha has disseminated through the physiology, it gets stuck in the ama, and this is how disease manifests.

Suppose then that a patient has a pitta imbalance, or vata imbalance, but digestion is strong; there is little or no ama, and the system is clean. That imbalanced dosha may cause the patient some symptoms, and may even prompt the patient to go to the physician. However, for this imbalanced dosha to manifest as more serious disease, it needs some ama to stick to. Ama serves as the substrate to which the imbalanced dosha binds to manifest disease. This helps clarify why in ayurveda we place such great emphasis on maintaining strong digestion. If we keep digestion strong, we keep the system clear of ama, and then for the most part we protect ourselves from serious illness. When talking about food and nutrition, then, the first thing a person needs to know is, how and when do we eat so as to assure that when we do so, we are nourishing ourselves rather than poisoning ourselves? How and when do we eat so as to support a strong digestive fire, promote the generation of ojas, and limit or eliminate the production of ama?

WHAT IS AMA?
According to ayurveda, "ama" represents the toxic byproduct of improperly or incompletely digested food. Although we have no similar concept in western medicine, one contemporary model may provide insight. Some scientists maintain that disruption of the lining of the intestine can lead to absorption of poorly digested food components.[9] This in turn triggers an immune response to the incompletely digested food molecules, leading to increased risk of systemic inflammatory diseases. It may be that these poorly digested food particles correlate with the concept of ama that has been a focus of ayurvedic therapeutics for generations.

The remainder of this chapter, and the next several chapters, will focus on nutrition and digestion. The material is of high importance, and as the above discussion suggests, these guidelines to proper digestion should be viewed as the cornerstone to the foundation of good health. Before we review these guidelines, however, let's consider the matter in the context of the medical and health concerns that patients commonly present with when seeking complementary and integrative care. According to ayurveda, most chronic pain conditions will have as at least a part of their cause weak digestion with ama accumulating in the part of the body that hurts. Weak digestion with ama accumulating in the muscles causes fibromyalgia in many patients. Osteoarthritis can often be attributed to weak digestion with ama accumulating in the joints. In such cases, ama accumulation isn't necessarily the whole story, but most of the time, it's at least part of the story. Any symptom along the lines of:

I'm tired all the time.

I have chronic pain.

I feel stiffness or achiness.

I'm fatigued.

I'm depressed.

I'm low on energy.

I have brain fog.

I have a sense of blockage in the physiology, or a sense that somehow things in the body aren't working quite right.

I experience frequent colds or respiratory infections.

All of these, according to ayurveda, can be attributed in many patients to ama accumulation. For almost all patients, the guidelines to proper digestion are highly important, relevant, and pragmatic.

The first thing that we are going to mention represents the most vital point we are going to make about food and nutrition. Let's make this the take-home message of these next few chapters. If you remember only one thing from this review, consider the following as the keypoint:

The main meal of the day should be at midday.

Lunch is the main meal. Dinner should be very light. The reason that you picked up this book was to learn simply this. Why is this point of such high importance? Remember we said that digestion, or "agni," is like a fire. When the sun is highest in the sky is when nature supports digesting the biggest meal of the day. According to ayurveda, digestion is naturally strongest at high noon. For that reason, 1600 kcal at lunch is way different from 1600 kcal at 8 p.m. Everything else we are going to say about food and nutrition is secondary to this. If you are going to do something you know you shouldn't do (like, for example, eating 3 pieces of pepperoni pizza), you are much more likely to get away with it if you do it at lunchtime as opposed to 8 p.m. In contrast, there is no such thing as a healthy, big meal at 8:00 at night, regardless of how pristine the ingredients. It is simply too late to be eating that much food. If someone is trying to lose a little weight, one of the first things we will tell him is to eat a little more for lunch, and reduce food intake at night. In other words, when and how we eat is as important as what we eat, and the answer to the question "When do we eat?" is midday, with a lighter dinner. Of all the stupid things that people do with food and nutrition in North America (which is, of course, quite a long list!), right up at the top, in terms of under-recognized causes, or aggravators, of a lot of common health problems is the habit that most people have of eating too heavily at night.

By this line of thinking, then, what is the worst possible time to eat those 3 pieces of pepperoni pizza? Midnight, with the sun on the opposite end of the earth, and your digestion tuned to its dead weakest. Think of your digestion as a gas stovetop, which is on high at noon, then burns lower and lower and lower until midnight, when it is nearly off; then higher and higher until noon, when it is back on high again.

Main meal midday, lighter dinner, breakfast is optional. Breakfast may not be optional for you, depending upon your lifestyle, habits, digestion, preferences, and so forth. There is no problem with eating a decent breakfast. The point is, some people come in to see us and comment, "Hey doc, when I wake up in the morning I don't feel like eating. I skip breakfast." This is not a problem. In contrast, other patients come in and say, "Hey doc, I'm a really busy guy at work during the day. I don't have time to eat lunch." Not okay. Skipping lunch runs counter to one's long-term prospects for maintaining good health.

The recommendation to eat your main meal at midday stems from ayurvedic theory as well as generations of clinical experience. In addition, emerging concepts and empiric data from contemporary biomedicine support this notion. We know that the human body has a "circadian clock" governing the function and rhythms of the physiology. (The term circadian refers to biological processes that occur naturally during a 24-hour cycle). The body's central timekeeper is located in a part of the brain known as the suprachiasmatic nucleus. Detection of light by the retina of the eye triggers the expression of circadian genes within the suprachiasmatic nucleus, which, in turn, regulate the sleep-wake cycle through the release of hormones such as cortisol, which triggers waking, as well as melatonin, which promotes sleep.

In addition to this central clock located in the suprachiasmatic nucleus of the brain, more recently it has been discovered that organs and tissues throughout the body are likewise controlled by circadian clocks of their own, regulated by circadian genes in their own cells.[10] For such internal organs, including the liver and gut, food intake represents an important signal as to the time of day. When food intake is timed to properly coincide with the light-dark cycle, the central and peripheral circadian clocks can work together in synchrony to achieve optimal metabolism. If, however, the peripheral clocks are thrown off, for example by eating heavily at night, this can result in discoordination of the central and peripheral clocks, leading to digestive and metabolic problems.

The idea that our digestive function is influenced by daytime light exposure is supported by experimental data. In one interesting study,[11] people exposed to dim light during the day, compared with those exposed to bright light, showed evidence of reduced carbohydrate absorption and stomach muscle electrical activity. Other data likewise support the traditional recommendation of eating the main meal during the day.[12,13] Scientists have shown that the speed of intestinal tract motility is higher during the day than at night. We also know that plasma insulin levels begin to rise in the morning, then peak in the afternoon, with a decline at night. In healthy people, the rise in plasma blood sugars after identical meals is higher at night than in the morning. The secretion of other digestive fluids has also been linked to the time of day. Saliva production is higher during the day than at night. In laboratory animals, the activity of digestive enzymes in the small intestine has been shown to be highest during periods of expected food intake; this rhythm persists during several days of fasting. In addition, in cross-sectional epidemiologic studies, scientists have shown an association between late-night eating and increased risk for heart disease, obesity, and metabolic syndrome.[14]

More research is needed in this area. Until then, current scientific data are consistent with the old ayurvedic concept that our digestive tract operates on a daily routine, and that patients can optimize digestive and metabolic health by eating their main meal at lunch.

No Grazing

Main meal midday, lighter dinner, breakfast optional. What about snacking? Snacking is perfectly fine, but grazing must be avoided. In other words, when we eat, we wait until the previous meal has been digested before eating again, which generally takes about 3 hours. If you had some oatmeal at 6:30 in the morning, and now it's 9:30 a.m. or 10 a.m., and you've been busy, and you're starving, and lunch isn't going to be until noon or 1 p.m., a piece of fruit or a handful of nuts is perfectly appropriate. But we don't graze, especially on junk.

As an analogy, suppose you start making some lentil soup, and you put the pot on the stovetop at 6 a.m., and toss in the lentils. Then at 7 a.m. you toss in some more lentils, and at 7:30 a.m. some more lentils, and at 8:30 a.m. some more lentils, and at 9:30 a.m. some more lentils, and at 10:00 a.m. again more lentils, then more lentils into the soup at 11 a.m., and so on, and then at noon you try serving it to someone. This meal is not going to be received well! Some of the lentils are overcooked, some undercooked, etc., and the dish may not even be edible. In the same way, if we are constantly grazing, especially on junk, the digestive processes are confounded with generation of ama. When you eat something, enjoy it! However, at some point you will to need to stop eating. As mentioned earlier, don't start eating again until what you have just consumed is digested, which usually takes about 3 hours.

When We Eat Is As Important As What We Eat

To summarize the routine as to when do we eat, the answer is midday lunch as the main meal, with a light dinner. Some of us just need to eat twice. Beyond that, a good, nutritious breakfast is a good idea if you like, as well as healthy midmorning snack, and/or a healthy midafternoon snack. That's it. We can eat those 5 times, but we shouldn't eat any more often than that. Of course, we never snack after dinner. Here as always, though, there can be exceptions. For example, if a patient has diabetes and is requiring insulin injections, the physician may advise the patient to have a snack before bedtime so the blood sugars don't go too low overnight. Unless your physician has specifically instructed you otherwise, NEVER snack after dinner. (Another important exception: A glass of warm milk with a pinch of cardamom or tumeric at bedtime is okay for most people).

One comment about breakfast. Some people like to have a heavy breakfast, and widely circulated rumors suggest that breakfast should be the main meal of the day. Although there is no problem with having a good breakfast, don't overdo it. If you have too much for breakfast, then you won't be so hungry for lunch. As a result, you'll be hungry at night, and may overeat at dinner, which is the big mistake we are trying to avoid.

Cold Drinks Are Off The Menu

Okay, now we get it. You must have your main meal at midday. Let's say you are at work, and you were too busy to make anything for your lunch, so you need to go out and find some healthy restaurant for your main meal. When you walk into virtually any restaurant in North America, what's the first thing you're served? Practically even before you have walked in the door, they've brought you ice water. Already we are off to a bad start! According to ayurveda, one should avoid iced beverages, especially with food. Room temperature beverages are fine, and warm beverages are actually beneficial. In other words, cold drinks are off the menu. Why must we avoid iced beverages, especially with food? Remember that digestion, or "agni," is like a fire. Anything cold extinguishes the digestive fire, whereas anything warm stimulates the fire. For this reason, according to ayurveda, we never drink cold anything. The next time a waiter or waitress brings you ice water, consider responding, "Sorry, no thank you, I'll take water with no ice." Or, for maximum results, the ambitious patient who wants to promote good health and wellness as expediently as possible can ask instead for plain hot water. "Tea without the tea bag."

Indeed, when we have a patient suffering from some medical problem related to weak digestion with ama accumulation (and remember, as previously suggested, probably 80% or so of chronic medical problems will have weak digestion with ama accumulation as at least part of their cause), we will send the patient off to the store to purchase a thermos. We then instruct the patient to fill the thermos with plain hot water, and to sip it throughout the day. Frequently sipping plain hot water heats up the digestive fire, melts away the ama, and provides a good, low-budget detoxification for just about anyone. You'll pay 20 bucks for the thermos, and then you are good to go for the next decade. As always, one shouldn't be extreme about this. If the temperature outside is 110 degrees Fahrenheit, and you wish to put some ice in your water to get it down to room temperature (70 or 75 degrees), this is of course perfectly fine. However, the general principle still stands: Don't drink cold anything!

Suppose you are on a camping trip, and you build a campfire. You work hard, it takes you about an hour, and now you have your campfire blazing. Then, just as you reach to put your potatoes in the fire, your kid or grandkid comes by and dumps a wheelbarrow full of ice on your campfire. This is not such a funny joke. Your potatoes aren't going to cook. In the same way, we avoid cold beverages in the diet.

Although experimental evidence in this area is lacking, we can speculate that the physiologic benefit of warm drinks versus cold can be potentially explained in several ways. Heat generally leads to dilation of blood vessels, which could improve intestinal blood flow during digestion. In addition, gut enzymatic activity may be facilitated, or enhanced, by warmer temperatures.

Cook Your Food

The same guideline that applies to beverages can be extended to food. As a general principle, we favor warm and well-cooked foods, because they are easier to digest. Likewise, we reduce or avoid cold and/or raw foods, which are harder to digest. The ayurvedic diet, then, is the *cooked food* diet. It is the 180-degree opposite of the raw food diet. We cook our food, then eat it warm, or at least room temperature. Cooking the food begins the process of digestion for us by breaking down the complex nutrients that we would otherwise need to digest on our own.[15] Fresh fruit has been cooked by the sun, so there is no need to cook your oranges or grapes. You can cook fresh fruit if you want to. For example, cooked apples or pears can make for a delicious breakfast or snack. However, as fruit has been cooked by the sun, you can eat berries right off the bush, apples right off the tree, or grapes right off the vine. Just about everything else, with one important exception (to be discussed later), you should cook first, and consume warm, or at least room temperature.

By this line of thinking, what is the most over-rated dish in the country in terms of its purported health-giving qualities? Salad. We should eat loads of vegetables, but they need to be cooked! We reduce or avoid raw vegetables, because they are hard to digest. We don't mind a little bit of salad as part of lunch, but certainly avoid eating a big salad at dinner time. Broadly speaking, vegetables are generally under-rated in the diet, but salad is way over-rated.

People commonly object that raw vegetables are more nutritious, because cooking the vegetables diminishes their nutritional content. Although it is true that when steaming your vegetables some of the water soluble nutrients may diffuse out, what remains is easier to digest and assimilate, hence the cooked vegetables effectively are more nutritious.

CROCKPOT APPLES

SERVES 2

Ingredients:

3-4 baking apples (gala, granny smith, etc.)

1 whole clove and/or ¼ tsp cinnamon

1 handful raisins (optional)

Variation: Another delicious option is to substitute pears for the apples, as per the above recipe.

Directions:

Wash and peel 3-4 baking apples. Core the apples, or just slice the flesh off the core. Place cored apples or apple slices into crockpot. (Discard the core.) Turn crockpot on low. Place 3 drops of water over the apples. Add a whole clove, and/or a pinch of ground cinnamon. You also have the option of adding a handful of raisins. Place cover on crockpot. Cook on low overnight, or for about 6 hours.

In the morning you will have satisfying, delicious homemade cooked apples ready for breakfast! This is especially good for balancing pitta dosha and for improving skin problems.

The Ideal Diet Is A Lactovegetarian Diet

According to ayurveda, the ideal diet is a lactovegetarian diet, i.e., a vegetarian diet that includes dairy products. Scientists have reported the many health benefits of a vegetarian diet in the medical literature, which include reduced risk for both cancer and cardiovascular disease.[16,17] Thus, adherence to a lactovegetarian diet is the ideal goal for most people. However, one does not necessarily need to be vegetarian to benefit from this program. If you are going to eat meat, poultry, fish, or eggs, have them at lunchtime. Eat only very small amounts, if any, meat products for dinner.

Although most people do not become fully vegetarian, a reason for mentioning vegetarianism is that, whereas we discourage eating too much in the way of salads, we do not want people to come away from this discussion thinking that we are telling you not to eat vegetables. To the contrary, the ideal diet is a lactovegetarian diet that should contain way more vegetables than most people in this culture even dream of. If you really try eating that many vegetables raw, you will quickly come around to understanding why it is recommended that you cook them. One might expect to experience too much in the way of gas, bloating, and other digestive challenges from a diet high in raw vegetable consumption.

What Should A Typical Day's Diet Look Like?

We'll start with breakfast. If you are going to have breakfast, what are some ideal breakfast items? Some cooked cereal, like oatmeal. Or, if your digestion is strong, a piece of toast with nut butter. Or, some stewed apples or pears (see recipe for Crockpot Apples).

When midmorning rolls along, if you need a snack, a piece of fruit or a handful of nuts would be ideal.

Now it's lunchtime, which will be your main meal of the day.

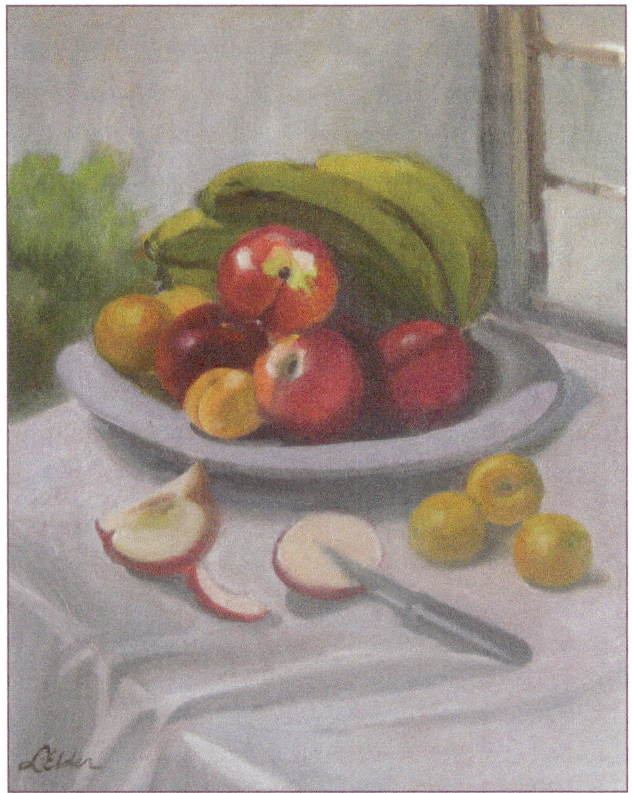

Cooked by the Sun

(oil on canvas)

After a trip to the spirited, open-air Mahane Yehuda market in central Jerusalem, we arranged the treasures gleaned for a portrait. What could be more lovely than white nectarines at their peak? Local fruit in season possesses an almost unearthly beauty, fragrance, and taste.

CHAPTER THREE

WHAT'S FOR LUNCH?

Recipes and menu options provide practical guidance for busy people who want to eat well.

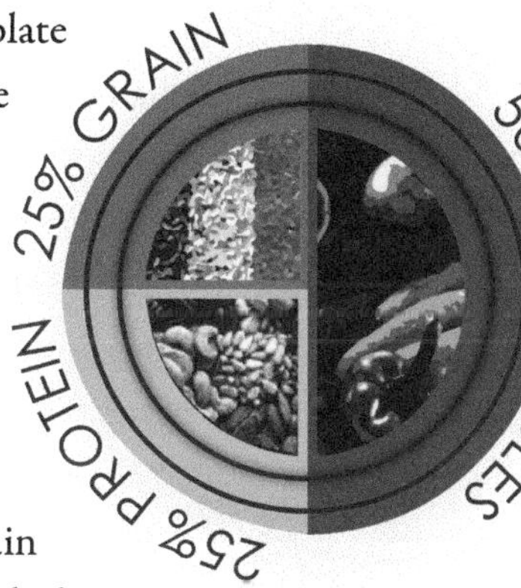

As the diagram shows, the biggest thing on the lunch plate should be a heap of cooked vegetables, filling up half the plate! Suppose you are having spinach as the vegetable selection. To fill half the plate at your biggest meal of the day with cooked spinach, you need to start with 3 or 4 bags of spinach, or more! This, of course, is considerably more than you would or could eat raw. The point is, we are talking about LOTS of vegetables.

25% GRAIN
50% VEGETABLES
25% PROTEIN

In addition to vegetables, we will include a whole grain (rice, pasta, millet, quinoa, rye, barley, couscous, buckwheat, bulgur wheat, amarynth, etc.) as well as some protein (beans, or whatever you are having, like tofu, poultry, fish, etc.). A piece of toast on the side, and there's your lunch!

As usual, the "devil is in the details." Although having a healthy main meal at lunch sounds like a simple idea, putting this into practice can be challenging, especially if this is a new idea for you, and/or if all the adults in your household are working. The remainder of this chapter focuses on fleshing out the details. How can we cook and eat in a healthy way in our busy, modern world? Below you will find recipes, cooking tips, meal options, and more!

VEGETABLES

Preparing Vegetables

You'll be eating loads of vegetables for lunch, and perhaps some for dinner as well. A little bit of salad at lunch is okay, especially in very hot weather, but for the most part the vegetables will be cooked. Let's review how to prepare the vegetables as part of a delicious, nutritious, easily digestible meal.

First, which vegetables are appropriate? Pick fresh vegetables that you will enjoy eating. As one example, a combination of kale, or another leafy green, with cabbage and carrots might be typical at lunchtime. As a general rule, lots of cooked leafy green vegetables are good for most people. In Chapter Five, we will review more about which vegetables are best to favor or avoid on the basis of which dosha must be balanced. In general, most vegetables, when properly cooked with spices and a little oil and then consumed at lunchtime, will be very well tolerated.

Before cooking vegetables, trim the ends of the stems and discard. For tougher greens such as kale and collards, remove the leaves and discard the woody stems. You can do this by "ribbing" the stems, or sliding your fingers firmly along the stems from the bottom to the top. Chard stems do not have to be removed and can be eaten along with the leaves.

Wash greens and other vegetables by immersing them in a large pan of water. Agitate, then lift them out and drain them in a colander. If needed, change the water, and repeat until the water is clean. Next, chop the vegetables (see Sidebar: Special Tip).

SPECIAL TIP:
Consider preparing vegetables for cooking in advance. In other words, you can wash, drain, and chop the vegetables when you have time and store them in large sealed plastic containers in your refrigerator for use over the next several days. If desired, chopped veggies that require longer cooking times, such as cabbage, collard greens, kale, green beans, and carrots, can be stored together in a container separate from veggies that are faster cooking (such as chopped chard, cauliflower, etc.). You will greatly speed the prep time for meals by having the vegetables ready to go. You can just dump the prepped veggies right into the steamer 5-10 minutes before serving.

Cooking Vegetables

Steam the vegetables, covered, in a steamer (a collapsible basket that you place in a covered pot with water at the bottom) until they are "fork-friendly." The vegetables should be easy to chew but not overcooked. Start denser vegetables, like string beans, kale, collards, carrots, and cabbage, first. Cook these for about 5-7 minutes. Next, add softer vegetables, like chard, cauliflower, and zucchini, and cook for about 5 minutes more. If using fast-cooking vegetables, such as spinach and asparagus, add to the steamer 1-2 minutes before removing the pan from the heat. Vegetables may then be spiced (next page) and eaten as is

SPICED STEAMED VEGETABLES — SERVES 2

Step 1:

For this dish, choose one or two types of leafy greens, and one or two types of other vegetables.

6-8 cups of chopped leafy greens; e.g., kale, collards, chard, mustard greens, or spinach (use twice as much spinach because it cooks down a lot).

2-4 cups of other vegetables; e.g., thinly sliced red or green cabbage, skinned and chopped carrots, 1-inch florets of cauliflower and/or broccoli, peeled and sliced daikon radish, finely cut green beans, or sliced asparagus.

Note: As a shortcut, if you don't have time to sauté the spices in the oil, you can just sprinkle a little ghee or olive oil onto the vegetables, and then sprinkle the dry spices onto the vegetables while they cook.

INDIAN-STYLE OPTION

Directions:

1. Steam vegetables, covered. Cook on medium-high heat for a total of about 10 minutes until vegetables are fork-friendly but not overcooked. Remove from heat.
2. Heat the ghee or olive oil in a small frying pan or medium saucepan. Gently sauté the whole spices (cumin seeds, fresh ginger, and mustard seeds) on medium-low heat while stirring, until the mustard seeds just start to pop (this generally takes a few minutes).
3. Remove the pan from the heat and stir in the ground spices: turmeric, optional ground coriander, and black pepper. (Ground spices only need to heat for a few seconds.) Lift the vegetables out of the steamer with a large spoon and roll them in the pan with the spiced oil before serving. You may squeeze some fresh lemon or lime juice on the vegetables before eating. Salt to taste.

Step 2.

2 tsp ghee (see Chapter Four) or olive oil
1 tsp cumin seeds
1 tsp peeled and diced fresh ginger
½ tsp black mustard seeds

Step 3.

½ tsp ground turmeric
1 tsp ground coriander (optional)
Pinch of ground black pepper
½ fresh lemon or lime juice (optional)
Salt

ITALIAN-STYLE OPTION

Directions:

1. Steam vegetables covered, as above.
2. Heat 2 tsp of olive oil in a small frying pan or medium-sized sauce pan, and add optional asafetida or garlic. Stir on medium-low heat for a minute. Add the Italian spices and stir for a few more minutes until fragrant. Remove from heat. Lift the vegetables out of the steamer with a large spoon and roll them in the pan with the spiced oil before serving.
3. Add black pepper. Salt to taste.

Steps 2 and 3.

2 tsp olive oil
Pinch of asafetida (see Note on page 32) or diced garlic (both are optional)
1 T of your choice of Italian spices such as dried basil, oregano, sage and thyme. If you are using fresh spices, use 3 times the amount because they are less potent.
Ground black pepper
Salt

or placed in a sturdy, tempered glass blender with the cooking water and blended with spices and a bit of oil to make a soup. Add salt to taste unless you are on a salt-restricted diet. Add pepper if desired.

Spicing Vegetables

Vegetables can be spiced according to any number of cuisines. Keep in mind that the use of spices is vital! Spices play a crucial role in helping us to properly digest and assimilate food. The addition of a little oil is also important for digestion and helps to activate the spices. See the recipes on page 31 for traditional spice combinations. These recipes are flexible to allow for selecting fresh seasonal vegetables.

NOTE:
Asafetida (hing) is the dried resin obtained from several plants native to India. It's good for digestion and substitutes for garlic and onions when added in small amounts to savory dishes. Asafetida boosts flavor without causing bad breath! Asafetida comes in various dilutions. The white variety is stronger and a few shakes is enough. The yellow variety can be used a little more liberally. It is activated by heating briefly in oil. You can find this spice in Indian food stores or through online sources.

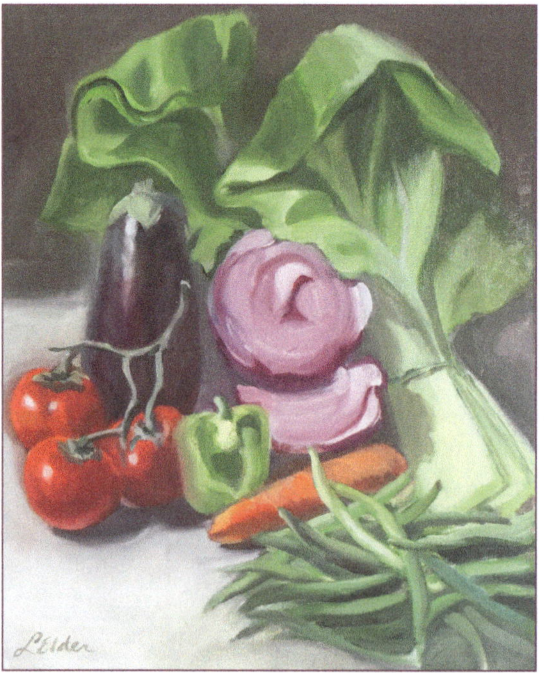

Preparing the Main Course
(oil on canvas)

Behold the supreme vitality and potential of these fresh vegetables, eagerly awaiting transformation into a cooked gourmet dish by the artful application of heat, spices, and a bit of oil. While shopping, pay attention to which vegetables and colors naturally draw you. Your body may be telling you what it needs.

GRAINS

In addition to vegetables, you will want to include a grain with your lunch. Grains are an important ayurvedic food. Enjoy grains with dal or bean dishes for an easy, satisfying meal. A combination of bulgur wheat, quinoa, and amaranth also makes a great cooked cereal for breakfast.

Which Grains?

According to ayurveda, grains with heavy husks, like rice and barley, are harder to digest, and therefore their pearled forms, e.g., white basmati rice and pearled barley, are recommended. Brown rice and barley with hulls are also fine for occasional use or for those with stronger digestion.

In general it's best to buy organic if possible; however, one exception is for aged, imported white basmati rice, available in Indian food stores but rarely labeled as organically grown. The quality of this rice, and the benefits of the aging process used, makes it a superior product to domestic organic basmati rice in the opinion of many.

If you have a kapha constitution, are trying to lose weight, or if it's kapha season, you might want to favor lighter grains that won't weigh you down. Barley, quinoa, rye, and amaranth are in this category. If you have a vata or pitta constitution, favor rice, and wheat products such as wheat berries, spelt, farro, bulgur wheat, and couscous. Refer to Chapter Five for a complete list of foods for specific constitutions.

Storing Grains

Store grains in a cool cabinet in glass jars, or plastic containers with tight-fitting lids to guard against moth infestation. When buying grains from a store you're not familiar with, putting the bags into the freezer for a few hours or overnight can ward off future infestations you might otherwise be bringing home.

Preparing Grains

Place the grain in a bowl, then rinse it with several changes of water, swishing it around with your fingers until the water is clear. This insures that the grain is clean and also, in the case of white rice and barley, gets rid of excess starch. For smaller grains, like amaranth and quinoa, it is helpful to pour off the rinse water through a fine sieve to avoid losing grain down the drain.

TASTY FAST-COOKING GRAINS — SERVES 2

Ingredients:

- ½ cup grain: choose one of the following: white basmati rice (imported, aged basmati rice is best—find it in Indian food stores, or online at amazon.com), quinoa, bulgur wheat, amaranth, couscous
- ¾ cup water
- 1 ½ tsp ghee or olive oil
- ¼ tsp salt
- 1 whole clove or dash of turmeric

These grains are good choices if you are short on time. Serve with bean or lentil (dal) dishes.

Directions:

Boil the water in a small pot and add the grain to the boiling water. Add the ghee or olive oil. Add the salt. Add the clove or turmeric.

Return to a boil, then reduce heat to low and simmer while covered for 15-20 minutes. Remove from heat and partially uncover. After 5 minutes, fluff with a fork and serve.

MELLOW SLOW-COOKING GRAINS — SERVES 2

Ingredients:

- ½ cup grain: choose one of the following: pearled barley, rye, spelt, farro, wheat berries, or brown rice
- 2 ½ - 3 cups water
- 1 T ghee or olive oil
- ¼ tsp salt
- 1 whole clove or dash of turmeric

These grains take a little longer to prepare but are nourishing and delicious, especially when served with dal and bean dishes.

Directions:

Boil the water in a small pot and add the grain to the boiling water. Add the ghee or olive oil. Add the salt. Add the clove or turmeric. Return to a boil, then reduce heat to low and simmer, covered, for 45-60 minutes, periodically stirring to prevent sticking, until grain is tender and fully cooked. You may add a little boiling water while cooking if the grain seems too dry. Wheat berries may take a little longer to cook than the others. Remove from heat and serve.

BEANS

Combining Legumes (Beans) And Grains

It's recommended to combine beans or lentils with a grain at lunchtime. The combination creates a satisfying and nutritious meal.

From a nutritional perspective, the combination of a legume and a grain provides for a "complete protein." What does this mean? Proteins are made up of building blocks called amino acids. In order to build the proteins needed by the body, there are a total of 10 amino acids that people require in the diet. Any food that provides all 10 of these required amino acids is considered a complete protein. Animal products, such as meats, eggs, and dairy products, are examples of foods that in and of themselves constitute complete proteins. Beans are good sources of protein, as are whole grains, but neither beans by themselves, nor grains by themselves, are complete proteins. That is to say, a legume, by itself, or a grain, by itself, will lack some of the 10 amino acids required by the body. However, when combined, the amino acids in the bean and the grain complement one another, and this combination will provide all of the 10 amino acids needed in the diet.

In many grocery stores, you will find a good selection of recommended grains and beans in the bulk section. Sometimes you can find free pamphlets with instructions for cooking each type of grain or bean.

Again, in all of these recipes, *the use of spices is very important!* Spices play an important role in helping us to properly digest and assimilate the food.

Guidelines For Cooking Beans

Beans have a reputation for causing gas and digestive problems, but by following a few simple guidelines, you can avoid this and take advantage of this amazing and economical protein source.

Larger beans, such as black beans and kidney beans, are best eaten at lunchtime because they are harder to digest. Pink lentils and brown lentils are easier to digest, but they are still best eaten at lunchtime, especially for those with a more delicate digestion.

For optimal digestibility, choose split mung dal. As the most digestible of the legumes, it's suitable for everyone, including those with delicate digestion, such as children, the elderly, and the ill. Urid dal and toor dal are also easy to digest. Dals can be found at Indian food stores, health food stores, or online through vendors like amazon.com.

Sort beans to remove foreign material, such as pebbles. This is not as much of a problem as it was in the past, but a quick inspection is still important to do.

Always rinse beans to remove the gas producing oligosaccharides. Soak those beans that require it. (See the section on soaking beans, page 36.)

Cook beans in fresh water. Never use the soaking water for cooking.

Simmer beans. Do not boil them. Boiling beans causes them to become tough.

Do not add cold water to beans while they are cooking because it disrupts the cooking process and may prevent the beans from softening. If needed, add boiling water.

Do not add salt or large amounts of acidic ingredients, like tomato or lemon juice, while the beans are cooking because it toughens the skins.

Give the beans enough time to cook. Undercooked beans are hard to digest. A slow cooker (crockpot) is great if you don't have the time or inclination to supervise a pot of beans for hours. A slow cooker allows you to safely cook a meal while you are away. Dals and pink lentils cook a lot faster than most of the beans and don't need to be soaked. They are good options for a faster cooking dish.

Soaking Beans: Which Ones Need It, Which Don't?

Many beans need to be soaked before cooking. Soaking helps rid beans of oligosaccharides, the main source of excessive gas production and digestive problems that some of them cause. It also shortens the cooking time. Beans that require soaking include black beans, garbanzo beans (chickpeas), kidney beans, white beans (such as navy and cannellini), and pinto beans.

Most lentils do not need to be soaked. These include brown lentils, French lentils, pink lentils, and green lentils. Mung, toor, and urid dals do not require soaking. Split peas do not require soaking.

For beans that require soaking, the required time is usually a minimum of 4 hours, or overnight. In a hurry? See the quick-soak shortcut below.

To soak, sort the beans and then place them in a bowl and cover with at least several inches of water.

When done soaking, drain and discard the soaking water, and cook with fresh water.

Quick Soak Shortcut

When you don't have time to soak beans for 4 hours or overnight, there's a faster way. Sort and rinse the beans, place them in a pot and cover with 2 inches of water. Bring water to boil and then turn off. Cover the pot and let it sit for 1 hour. Drain and discard soaking water and cook beans as directed.

SPLIT MUNG DAL

SERVES 2

Split mung dal is the most easily digestible legume and is highly recommended in ayurvedic cuisine as an important protein source. This dish balances all three doshas. You can find the tiny yellow lentils in bags or in bulk at local health food stores or Indian food stores. The following recipe makes a soothing yet nourishing soup. You can vary the ratio of water to beans to make the dal thinner or thicker according to your tastes. Serve with a cooked grain.

Directions:

1. Clean the dahl. Boil water in a pot and add the dal. Return to a boil, reduce heat to low, and simmer until the dal is tender, 45 minutes to 4 hours, depending on the type of dal used. Split mung dal takes about 45 minutes to 1 hour to cook.
2. While the dal is cooking, place the ghee or olive oil into a small saucepan. Sauté the spices over medium-low heat in the saucepan. The spices need close supervision so they do not burn. Add the fresh ginger, cumin seeds, mustard seeds, and asafetida, if using. Sauté the spices for 1-3 minutes, while stirring, until the cumin and ginger darken a bit or until the mustard seeds start to pop. Remove from heat. Add the ground turmeric to the spice mixture.
3. When the dal is tender, add the spice mixture. Add the salt, pepper, and sweetener, if using. Whisk the dal until smooth. Cook a few minutes longer for the flavors to blend. Stir in cilantro just before serving.

Step 1.

½ cup split mung dal (you can also use urid dal, pink dal, split peas, or brown or green lentils)
3 cups water (more water may be added toward the end of cooking if it seems too thick)

Steps 2 and 3.

1 T ghee or olive oil
1 T fresh ginger, peeled, then grated or diced
1 tsp cumin seeds
½ tsp black mustard seeds
Pinch of asafetida (optional)
½ tsp turmeric
¼ tsp sugar or a pinch of stevia (optional)
Ground black pepper
Salt
2 T chopped fresh cilantro (optional)

KHICHARI — SERVES 2-3

Step 1.

½ cup basmati rice (the most digestible is aged white basmati rice)
⅓ cup split mung dal. Toor dal, lentils, or split peas could also be substituted
2 ½ cups water

Steps 2 and 3.

1 T ghee or olive oil
1 T grated or diced fresh ginger
¾ tsp cumin seeds
½ tsp mustard seeds
¼ tsp ground fenugreek seeds; whole seeds can be ground in your blender or used as they are
1 tsp turmeric
Salt
Several pinches of sugar or stevia (optional)
¼ cup chopped fresh cilantro (optional)

An important dish in ayurvedic cuisine, split mung bean khichari balances all three doshas. This is the optimal dish for those with delicate digestion, those recovering from an illness, and for children and the elderly. The following recipe for khichari makes a nutritious and soothing staple that provides a complete protein at lunch.

Directions:

1. Clean the rice and dal. In a medium pot boil the fresh water. Add the rice and dal, return to a boil, then reduce the heat to low. Cover the pot and simmer for 45 minutes to an hour, until the dal is tender, and all of the water is absorbed. The mixture will be quite thick. Stir occasionally and monitor closely towards the end to make sure it's not sticking. Add water if needed.
2. Meanwhile, in a small saucepan, heat the ghee or olive oil on medium low heat. Add the ginger, cumin, mustard seeds and fenugreek. Stir until the mustard seeds pop, then remove from heat. Add the turmeric.
3. When the rice and dal are well cooked, remove from heat and uncover. Add spices. Whisk until very smooth. Add salt and optional sweetener.

Optional:

Garnish with cilantro a few minutes before serving.

SMART LUNCHES: AYURVEDIC SLOW COOKER RECIPES

Slow Cooker

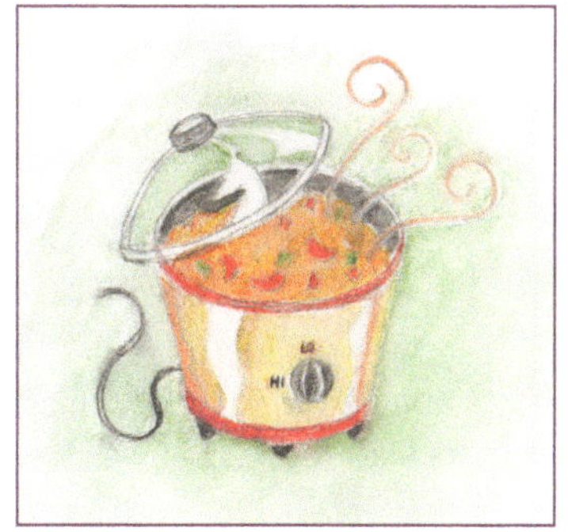

The slow cooker is a glorious thing for busy cooks. The beauty of the slow cooker, or crockpot, is that you can put beans, grain, and a bit of oil into the slow cooker before bed, let it cook all night, and then have a hot meal to put into a thermos in the morning to take to work. Because spices and vegetables easily overcook, it's best to put them in the slow cooker about an hour or so before leaving for work in the morning. To save time in the morning, you can measure the spices and cut up raw, slow-cooking vegetables (e.g., carrots, sweet potatoes, kale or collard greens) the day or night before. Set these aside in a sealed plastic container, and then dump them into the slow cooker along with spices, salt, and pepper about an hour before you pack your thermos in the morning.

The following hot lunch recipes are specifically designed to be made in a slow cooker but can also be prepared on the stove. You can find all different types of slow cookers on the market. Smaller sizes are ideal for a single person or couple. You don't need anything fancy, and a basic one with a low and high setting is perfect. We usually just use the low setting on our slow cooker, but the settings may vary with different brands.

Thermoses

If you are packing a hot lunch to take with you to work, you will need a good thermos or two. Wide-mouthed stainless steel, vacuum-sealed types are great because they keep food very hot and are durable: They don't break when dropped. Food in a vacuum-sealed thermos will continue to cook a bit for a few hours. A stainless steel thermos can be placed upside down in the lower rack of a dishwasher for cleaning. Don't put the cap in the dishwasher, though, as this will shorten its lifespan. It's nice but not mandatory to preheat your thermos by filling it a third of the way with boiling water, then sealing it with the cap for a few minutes. Then, unseal it, discard the water, scoop the food into the thermos with a large serving spoon, and seal it back up. Don't forget to pack a fork, spoon, napkin, and bowl with the thermos. You will be eating like royalty!

HEARTY LENTIL STEW

SERVES 2-3

Step 1.

⅓ cup lentils
⅓ cup pearled barley, rye, farro, wheat berries, brown rice, or other slow cooking grain
2 ½ cups water
2 tsp olive oil

Step 2.

1 small chopped tomato (optional)
1 tsp cumin seeds
1 tsp dried thyme
Pinch of asafetida (may substitute 1 small clove minced garlic if you can't get asafetida)
Pinch of crushed chili pepper (optional)
Salt
Ground black pepper
2 cups chopped slow-cooking vegetables like kale, collards, sweet potatoes and/or carrots

Note: For kale and collard greens, remove the leaves from the tough stems, discard stems and chop the leaves finely so that they will cook fully. Cut sweet potatoes into small cubes. Slice carrots into rings.

You can use regular brown lentils. Small French green lentils, if you can get them, are especially good.

Directions:

1. Clean the lentils and grain. Add fresh water to the bowl that contains the lentils and grain and pour the mixture into a slow cooker or stovetop cooking pot. Add oil.
2. Follow directions for your cooking method below:

Slow cooker directions:

Cook on the low setting with the lid on for 6 hours or overnight.

In the morning when you wake up, check the stew. Add a little hot water if it seems dry. Turn the crockpot to the high setting, add all of the rest of the ingredients, stir well, and cover. If you have premeasured the spices and prepped the vegetables the night before, this takes just a minute.

Continue to cook on the high setting for 30 minutes to 1 hour more or until the vegetables are fork friendly and the lentils are tender. Spoon the stew into the prepared thermos, close the cap firmly, and it's ready to go!

Stovetop directions:

Bring the stew to a boil, then reduce the heat and gently simmer, partially covered, on low for about 2 hours or until the grains and lentils are tender, stirring a few times to prevent sticking. You can add extra water if needed.

Turn the heat up to medium-low and add the spices and vegetables, stir well, and partially cover. Continue cooking until the vegetables are fork friendly, about 30 minutes, then serve immediately, or remove from heat and reheat for serving later.

ZESTY SPLIT PEA SOUP WITH CARROTS

SERVES 2-3

A refreshing ayurvedic take on conventional split pea soup.

Directions:

1. Clean the peas and grain. Add the specified amount of fresh water to the bowl that contains the peas and grain and pour the mixture into a slow cooker or stovetop cooking pot on the stove. Add the oil.
2. Follow directions for your cooking method below:

Slow cooker directions:

Cook with the lid on for 6 hours or overnight on low.

Stovetop directions:

Bring the soup to a boil in the pot, then reduce heat and simmer on low, partially covered, for about 3 hours until peas are soft, stirring a few times to prevent sticking. Add extra water if needed.

For both slow cooker and stovetop cooking:

When the peas are done, whisk briskly until somewhat smooth. The grains will give some texture to this dish. Add the cumin seeds, asafetida if using, fresh ginger, turmeric, salt and pepper directly to the soup. Whisk again. Add the carrots, cover, and cook another 15-30 minutes. Then, using a large spoon or ladle, spoon the stew into a prepared thermos or serve as desired. Garnish with fresh cilantro before serving (optional).

Step 1.

⅓ cup split peas
⅓ cup pearled barley, rye, spelt, farro, wheat berries, brown rice, or other slow cooking grain
3 cups water
2 tsp olive oil

Step 2.

½ tsp cumin seeds
Pinch of asafetida (optional)
2 tsp fresh grated or diced ginger root
½ tsp turmeric
Salt
Ground black pepper
1 large carrot, sliced in rings
¼ cup chopped fresh cilantro (optional)

ITALIAN WHITE BEAN SOUP WITH SAGE

SERVES 2-3

Step 1.

⅓ cup dried small navy beans (follow the directions on page 36 to presoak the beans)
⅓ cup barley, rye, spelt, farro, wheat berries, brown rice, or other slow-cooking grain
2 cups water
1 ½ tsp olive oil

Step 2.

1 ½ tsp more olive oil
2 T chopped fresh sage
Several pinches of asafetida (1 clove minced garlic may be substituted)
1 T sun-dried tomatoes, chopped (optional)
1 medium tomato, chopped (optional)
Salt
Ground black pepper
Juice from ¼ fresh lemon

Don't try substituting dried sage, it's just not the same! Envision yourself strolling through a field of sage in Tuscany. Delicious served with Lemony Vegan Pesto as a garnish (see page 45). If you soak the beans with a leaf of the sage, it enhances the flavor.

Directions:

1. Clean and soak the beans. Discard soak water. Clean the grain. Place soaked beans and grain into a medium bowl. Add the water to the mixture and pour into a slow cooker or stovetop cooking pot . Add 1 ½ tsp olive oil.
2. Follow directions for your cooking method below:

Slow cooker directions:

Cook in the slow cooker with the lid on for 6 hours or overnight on low.

Stovetop directions:

Bring the mixture to a boil in a pot on the stove, then reduce heat and gently simmer on low for about 3 hours, partially covered, stirring a few times to prevent sticking. You can add additional water if it seems dry.

For both slow cooker and stovetop cooking:

When the stew is almost done, heat on low another 1 ½ tsp olive oil in a small saucepan on stove. Add the asafetida or garlic to the oil, and sauté while stirring for 1 minute on medium-low heat. Add the chopped fresh sage and optional sun-dried tomatoes; stir for another few minutes. Add the optional fresh tomatoes, raise the heat to medium, and stir constantly until the tomatoes are soft and the kitchen is aromatic. Remove from heat. Ten minutes before the stew is done, add spice mixture, as well as the salt and pepper. Squeeze in lemon juice. Using a large spoon or ladle, spoon the stew into a prepared thermos or serve as desired.

GARBANZO AND POTATO INDIAN STEW

SERVES 2

The sesame oil, ground coriander, cilantro, and lemon combine to create a saucy broth in this fragrant dish. Make sure you use cold-pressed, natural sesame oil, not the chemically processed kind.

Directions:

1. Clean and soak the beans. Discard soak water. Clean the grain. Add the specified amount of water to the mixture and pour it all into a slow cooker or stovetop cooking pot. Add sesame oil.
2. Follow directions for your cooking method below:

Slow cooker directions:

Cook in a slow cooker with the lid on for 6 hours or overnight on low.

Stovetop directions:

Bring the stew to a boil in a pot on the stove, reduce heat, and gently simmer on low for about 3 hours, partially covered, stirring a few times to prevent sticking. You can add additional water if the stew seems dry.

For both slow cooker and stovetop cooking:

30 minutes to 1 hour before the stew is done, add the potato. Heat the remaining oil (1 ½ tsp) on low in a small saucepan on the stove. Place the cumin seeds and optional asafetida into the pan and turn it up to medium-low heat, stirring for a few minutes. Remove from heat and add the turmeric, ground coriander, and optional cayenne to the pan. When the stew is done, stir the spice mixture into it. Add the salt and pepper and squeeze in the lemon juice. Stir to combine.

Using a large spoon or ladle, spoon the stew into a prepared thermos or serve as desired. Garnish with cilantro before serving. If you are using a thermos, chopped cilantro can be brought along in a small separate plastic container so it doesn't overcook in the thermos.

Step 1.

½ cup uncooked garbanzo beans—also called chickpeas (follow presoak directions on page 36)
½ cup barley, rye, spelt, farro, wheat berries, brown rice, or other slow-cooking grain
3 cups water
1 ½ tsp cold-pressed sesame oil

Step 2.

1 small red new potato, cut into small cubes (it's not necessary to peel it)
Another 1 ½ tsp cold-pressed sesame oil
1 tsp cumin seeds
Several pinches of asafetida (optional)
½ tsp turmeric
1 ½ tsp ground coriander seeds
Dash of cayenne pepper (optional)
Salt
Ground black pepper
Juice from ½ lemon
¼ cup chopped fresh cilantro as garnish

WHY FRESH GINGER? AN EASY WAY TO KEEP IT ON HAND

Fresh ginger is a vital spice in ayurveda. It is considered to be a rasayana, a spice that is beneficial for most everyone. In fact, ayurveda refers to ginger as "the universal medicine." Ginger stimulates digestion without aggravation. It adds a pleasing punch and heat to many dishes without causing heartburn, as chilis can do.

Fresh ginger is available in the produce section of most supermarkets. Ideally, try to find the type with long, straighter branches because it's easier to prepare.

To prepare ginger: Rinse and cut off a branch a few inches long or more. Peel with a potato peeler or paring knife. Cut the branch into a few smaller chunks and place them into a food processor with a steel blade. Pulse several times until ginger is minced. If you don't have a food processor, you can mince it with a sharp knife or grate it with a grater. Store in a small, sealed jar in the refrigerator for up to 3 to 4 days. You can add a pinch of ginger to milk before warming it to drink, or to the cooking water when making cooked cereals. Add ginger to oil when sautéeing spices for vegetables or dals. You can even add a thin slice of ginger to boiling water for a cup of ginger tea or use it in Spicy Milk (see recipe in Chapter Four).

If you are in a pinch and can't obtain fresh ginger, 1 teaspoon fresh minced ginger equals ¼ teaspoon dry ground ginger. Be aware that dry ginger can have a drying effect on the colon and doesn't have the same beneficial effects as fresh.

GARNISHES

Here are 2 recipes that can serve as tasty garnishes at lunchtime.

GREEN SAUCE — SERVES 4 OR MORE

- 1 large handful fresh cilantro (fresh dill can be substituted)
- 1 large handful fresh parsley
- ¼ cup grated unsweetened coconut
- ¼ cup water
- Juice from 1 lemon
- 1 tsp salt
- Dash of cayenne pepper (optional)

This sauce is tridoshic, or balancing for all of the doshas. Everyone seems to love it, even kids! Green sauce enhances digestion but must be eaten the same day it's made. This is great as a topping on dal dishes, cooked veggies, or pasta. If you are craving fresh dill, you can substitute it for the cilantro for a delicious variation.

Directions:

Wash the cilantro and parsley, drain and place into a food processor with a steel blade. Add the coconut, water, lemon juice, salt, and optional cayenne. Pulse a few times until medium texture.

Place in a small covered container and serve the same day.

LEMONY VEDIC PESTO

SERVES 4 OR MORE

1 large handful fresh basil (large stems removed)
1 large handful fresh parsley
¼ cup pine nuts, walnuts, or unsalted almonds
½ cup nutritional yeast (available in health food sections of larger supermarkets)
Lemon zest from 1 lemon (optional) With a microplane this takes 10 seconds, or use a potato peeler—peel off just the outer part of the peel (not the bitter white part) and slice the peel finely with a sharp knife
Juice from 1 lemon
½ cup olive oil + 1 T extra oil if using asafetida
Several pinches of asafetida or 1 clove peeled and minced garlic

Try this vegan pesto as a topping or garnish on lentil or bean stews, pasta, or cooked vegetables. It's also great on bread or crackers. It's best fresh but can be stored for several days in a sealed container in the refrigerator. Adding lemon zest kicks it up a notch.

Directions:

Wash basil and parsley, drain in colander, then roll in tea towel or paper towel to dry. Place the basil, parsley, nuts, nutritional yeast, optional lemon zest, and lemon juice into a food processor with a steel blade. Add ½ cup olive oil and garlic if using. If you are using asafetida, it must be activated by heat. To do this, place 1 T of olive oil and the asafetida into your smallest saucepan. I actually just carefully hold a stainless steel measuring cup by its long handle an inch above the burner to do this. Heat on medium for a minute until the oil just starts to form tiny bubbles, and you see the asafetida powder sizzle slightly for a few seconds. Remove pan from heat and add the mixture to the food processor.

Pulse mixture several times to get a medium, but not completely smooth, texture.

Store in covered container until served.

There's your lunch! There are many more ideas, but we have included enough recipes to get you started with a good variety of delicious, healthy, nutritious meals.

Now it's midafternoon. If you need a snack, a piece of fruit or a handful of nuts would be ideal. Next, dinner time. Your dinner can look just like your lunch, except much less quantity, especially for the grain and the protein. Another good dinner option would be some cereal, like oatmeal with warm milk. Or, just warm milk and herbal tea.

Finally, what about the evening snack? Trick question! There's no evening snack. After dinner, we are done eating for the day!

CHAPTER FOUR

GLUTEN, DAIRY, AND A FEW MORE SURPRISES

Answers to some of the most commonly asked questions about food and nutrition.

Is It Okay To Eat Gluten?

Gluten is a protein found in some grains. Currently a lot of people are focused on avoiding gluten in the diet to improve health. It's true that some people cannot tolerate gluten, but gluten is fine for most people.

Celiac disease is a condition in which consumption of gluten triggers an inflammatory reaction of the lining of the small intestine. This leads to poor absorption of nutrients, diarrhea, excess gas, foul smelling stools, abdominal discomfort, and other symptoms. The incidence of celiac disease has increased dramatically in recent years and is thought to be in the range of 1%.[18] Physicians can often diagnose celiac disease using a simple blood test, and symptoms respond well to a gluten-free diet. Thus people who have celiac disease must avoid eating gluten. This can be accomplished by avoiding grains that contain gluten (like wheat, rye, and barley). Other grains, like rice and quinoa, do not contain gluten, and are fine for people with celiac disease to include in the diet.

Although people who have celiac disease must avoid gluten, for most other people, eating gluten is perfectly appropriate. Certain individuals without celiac disease may have some level of intolerance to gluten, but this remains controversial and poorly understood.[19,20] Many people who do not have celiac disease report feeling better after eliminating gluten from the diet. This could possibly be caused by a low-level gluten intolerance of some type, but it could also be explained by a number of potential confounders. First, when people decide to go gluten free, they typically start reading labels, and taking more care in selecting what foods they buy. They begin to reduce or eliminate junk foods, and start feeling a lot better. This improvement might simply be because they are generally eating healthier, having nothing at all to do with gluten. Secondly, given the near hysteria in the public consciousness surrounding gluten, some power of persuasion, or "placebo effect," may be at play.

Bear in mind also that foods containing gluten frequently also contain a type of carbohydrate called "fructans." Recent research suggests that the gastrointestinal symptoms experienced by patients self-reporting a diagnosis of gluten sensitivity may be caused not by gluten, but rather by the fructans.[21] In one study, the investigators gave participants muesli bars containing either fructans, gluten, or placebo. Those consuming the fructan-containing bars reported significantly worse gastrointestinal symptoms compared with those consuming the gluten. There was no significant difference between gluten and placebo.

If steering clear of gluten makes you feel better, it is no problem to continue doing so. Nevertheless, grains such as bulgur wheat, rye, and barley are extremely healthy foods for most people. Although these grains contain gluten, when consumed as freshly cooked whole grains, they can constitute an important part of a balanced and nutritious diet and will be well tolerated by the great majority of individuals. Such grains have been staple foods across multiple cultures for millennia. In the thousands-year-old tradition of ayurvedic dietary therapeutics, there are no concerns specified with regard to gluten-containing grains.

If you have celiac disease, you must eliminate gluten from your diet. If you do not have celiac disease, you can still reduce or eliminate gluten in the diet if you feel it improves your situation, but much of the time it may not be necessary.

What About Dairy Products?

Dairy products are a perfect food, or a perfect disaster, depending upon whether you follow a few rules. Ayurveda provides one set of guidelines for milk, another set of rules for cheese and yogurt, then another set of guidelines for butter. For milk (cow's milk, goat's milk), there are two important things to know. First, milk must be a hot beverage, and should not be consumed cold. Specifically, milk should be heated just to the point of boiling and then consumed hot or warm. When you see small bubbles forming on top of the hot milk, that's when it's time to take it off the heat. You can then let it cool down a bit as desired. If your milk has been pasteurized, boil it anyway. Boiling takes the milk to a higher temperature than routine pasteurization. It "denatures," or unwinds the protein molecules, making it easier to digest. Cold milk can be hard to digest, and may be kapha aggravating (i.e., it might be expected to cause increased congestion). By bringing the milk to boiling before consuming it, we significantly neutralize these issues. For even better effect, add a slice of fresh ginger or a pinch of turmeric to the milk as you heat it. The second rule is milk can only be combined with sweet-tasting foods. We cannot combine milk with bitter, sour, salty, pungent, or astringent foods. We'll consider grains to be sweet. You can combine milk with breakfast-style foods, e.g., a piece of toast or some cereal, or you can combine milk with dessert or with a cookie. On the other hand, you wouldn't want to combine milk with lunch or dinner. That is to say, you shouldn't combine milk with your tuna sandwich or your lasagna.

To summarize, milk brought just to boiling and consumed hot, by itself, or with something sweet is an ideal beverage, constituting an important and nutritious component of a vegetarian diet. In contrast, cold milk out of the refrigerator with your chicken stir-fry is not such a great idea and can lead to congestion, ama accumulation, and digestive challenges. The great majority of people who report difficulty digesting milk products, including those with lactose intolerance, actually can tolerate milk just fine in moderate amounts,[22] with the ability to do so greatly enhanced simply by adhering to these two rules. Heating milk has been shown to reduce allergenicity[23] and studies have demonstrated that the great majority of children with milk allergy can tolerate milk if heated.[24]

In addition, milk affords an exception to the "never snack after dinner" rule. If you need to have something at night, a cup of boiled milk, with a little cardamom and/or sweetener, provides a healthy bedtime snack.

What about soy milk or almond milk? These are not dairy products and are not the subject of our discussion. If you wish to use them, remember not to drink them cold. However, the concern about food combinations would not apply. Remember that these are processed beverages, so be sure to look at the label to check for healthy ingredients.

In summary, many people have concerns about milk, but most of the time such concerns are misplaced. Used and prepared properly, milk can be a delicious and important part of the diet. Most people who have milk allergies or lactose intolerance will tolerate milk just fine, if consumed according to the guidelines outlined above. In contrast, cold milk out of the refrigerator with your lunch, or a bowl of ice cream after dinner every night, are recipes for trouble.

Although the improper use of milk can cause congestion, the proper use of milk can actually provide therapeutic benefit for patients with congestion or respiratory symptoms. See the recipe for spicy milk on page 50, which provides a delicious nourishing and therapeutic drink to those suffering from respiratory symptoms.

Spicy Milk

(watercolor)

Ayurveda prescribes "Spicy Milk" as a therapeutic hot drink to reduce congestion. Always heat milk just to boiling before drinking, and take milk alone or with sweet foods like toast or cereal. Purchase the freshest milk you can find—check the expiration date on the container. Milk is extolled in ayurveda as a highly beneficial food, having a bliss-producing effect on consciousness.

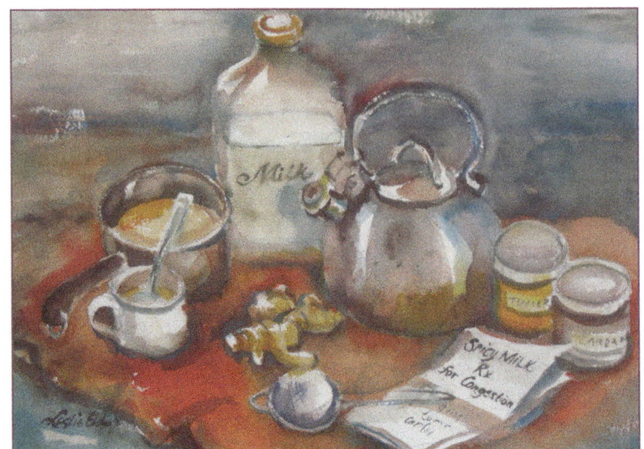

SPICY MILK

Ingredients:

1 cup water
1 slice of fresh raw ginger (ground ginger dries the colon and is not preferred)
(¼ tsp fresh ground pepper may be substituted for the ginger)
½ tsp turmeric
½ tsp cardamom
1 cup of milk

Directions:

Boil the water. Add the spices. Reduce heat and simmer for 2 minutes. Add milk, and bring to boil. Remove from heat, strain into a cup and enjoy! (You can add a small amount of cane sugar or stevia to taste if desired).

In contrast to milk, cheese and yogurt are okay to have with lunch. In fact, as these are heavier foods, lunch is the preferred time. Fresh cheeses, i.e., the "wet" cheeses, are much better for you than aged cheeses. When we say that cheese can be a healthy and nourishing food, we are talking about cottage cheese, panir, fresh mozzarella, etc. These would be healthier than, say, an aged cheddar.

Yogurt is an important food that is best consumed in the middle of the day. The preferred way to have yogurt is to make lassi, a simple and nutritious yogurt drink (see recipe for Lassi). Lassi should be considered a staple in the diet, ideally consumed daily after lunch.

Among the benefits of lassi is that it provides probiotic support. What does this mean? Scientists are showing increased interest in and awareness of the importance of maintaining the health of the "microbiome."[25] This term refers to the large number of health-promoting bacteria and other microorganisms that normally inhabit the human intestinal tract. Maintaining the right balance of healthy bacteria in the gut is increasingly understood as playing an important role in digestion and overall health. Lassi and other yogurt products contain helpful bacteria that are supportive of health and digestion. We can think of lassi as a "natural probiotic." Drinking lassi on a regular basis is a good way to promote the health of the microbiome.

We do not encourage the use of a lot of butter. Ghee, which is made from butter, is

LASSI

Directions:

Combine 1 part yogurt with 2-3 parts water. To make sweet lassi, add a little sweetener to taste. For salty (also called "spicy") lassi, instead add a pinch of salt and a pinch of cumin. Blend the ingredients together and enjoy! Remember to consume lassi at room temperature, never cold.

Ingredients:

Yogurt (homemade, or plain organic)
Water
Either sweetener (like cane sugar or stevia) to make sweet lassi, or salt + cumin to make salty lassi

GHEE

Directions:

Heat butter in slow cooker on low for about 14-16 hours, depending on your particular slow cooker. You should start with at least 2 lbs of butter. The ghee is ready when the butter has turned a clear golden yellow. The bottom of the pot will be medium to dark brown and very firm, allowing you to pour off the clear golden ghee easily, leaving the debris at the bottom behind. If the debris at the bottom is still clear and liquidy, cook it for another hour or two. Strain the ghee (the clear yellow fluid on top) through a cheese cloth or fine-mesh metal strainer into jars. An easy way to do this is to first place a large glass measuring cup or pot with a pouring spout into the sink. Place a large fine mesh metal strainer or some cheesecloth over the cup or pot. Pour a large amount of your ghee through the strainer into it, then remove the strainer. Place a jar into the sink and place a strainer or more cheesecloth over the jar mouth. Pour the hot ghee from the measuring cup or pot into the jar. Discard the debris at the bottom of the crockpot. Seal jars with lids and store at room temperature for up to 3 months. Do not refrigerate ghee because it renders the ghee less wholesome.

Ingredients:

Unsalted organic butter, at least 2 pounds

Materials:

Slow cooker
Several widemouth jars
Fine-mesh metal strainer or cheesecloth

a much better option (see recipe for Ghee). Ghee contains a healthier balance of fats compared with regular butter.[15] You can use ghee on your toast, or as an ideal cooking oil. (Other favorable cooking oils include olive oil for low to medium-heat cooking, as well as safflower oil, sunflower oil, and organic canola oil.)

Is It Better To Go Vegan?

Vegan diets have become increasingly popular. A vegan diet is a vegetarian diet that excludes all animal products, including dairy products and eggs. Another phrase in common use is "plant-based diet." This phrase means different things to different people. For some, "plant-based" refers to a diet that focuses on plant products, but allows for limited amounts of animal products, including meat, preferably fish or chicken. For others, "plant-based diet" denotes a strict vegan diet that not only completely excludes dairy products but also eliminates most oils as well.

In ayurveda, as a general principle we favor a lactovegetarian diet. As already noted, this is a vegetarian diet that includes dairy products. We take a more nuanced approach to dairy products. As outlined above, dairy products can be really good, or really bad, depending upon how you use them. The ayurvedic lactovegetarian diet has evolved over millenia, is nutritious and sustainable, is nutritionally complete,[26] and has withstood the test of time. Veganism has recently become popular but is incomplete nutritionally. Specifically, the vegan diet is deficient in vitamin B_{12}. If you are going to follow such a diet, it is important that you take a B_{12} supplement (about 1 mg a day orally is appropriate). B_{12} is an important vitamin found in animal (including dairy) products only. If someone adheres strictly to a vegan diet, over an extended period, without B_{12} supplementation, that individual can become deficient in the vitamin, leading to a condition called pernicious anemia. This is a serious and potentially fatal disease. Scientists isolated and identified Vitamin B_{12} as the deficient factor in pernicious anemia in the late 1940s, so it would not have been possible to purchase B_{12} supplements before then. That is to say, only in recent decades has it been possible for a population to safely consider this diet on a sustained basis. Other micronutrients that may be lacking in the vegan diet include calcium and long-chain omega 3 fatty acids.[27] A vegan diet, with B_{12} supplementation, is a fantastic improvement over the typical American diet and may be of benefit to many patients. However, this diet is clearly not for everyone and is certainly not the diet our species evolved to eat. A lactovegetarian diet, in contrast, is complete and requires no supplementation.

Many people find a vegan diet to be too difficult to sustain long term. The lactovegetarian diet is less restrictive, and thus easier to maintain. In the context of a vegetarian diet, dairy products can represent an important source of dietary nutrients, including protein, calcium, and, as stated, the main source of vitamin B_{12}. In addition, lassi provides important probiotic support. Finally, ayurveda details two additional reasons to include dairy products in a vegetarian diet. First, a strictly vegan diet can aggravate vata dosha. Second, dairy products, properly prepared, are considered "sattvic" foods (see Sidebar: How Does What You're Eating Affect Your Mind?), and it is important to emphasize such foods in the diet.

In summary, the lactovegetarian ayurvedic diet has evolved over a period of many centuries, and represents the collective wisdom and experience of multiple generations. Both scientific research and generations of clinical experience have shown this diet to be health promoting and sustainable. The vegan diet represents a tremendous improvement over the typical Western diet, but may be more difficult to sustain and is incomplete nutritionally. If you are going to stick with a vegan diet, be sure to take a vitamin B_{12} supplement.

HOW DOES WHAT YOU'RE EATING AFFECT YOUR MIND?

In ayurveda, we can classify foods into 3 types on the basis of the impact the food has on the mind. At this level, the 3 types of foods are *sattvic, rajasic*, and *tamasic*.

Sattvic foods have an evolutionary impact on the mind, and promote mental clarity, successful personal growth, forward progress in life, and transcendence in meditation practice. Examples of sattvic foods include: basmati rice, mung dal, fresh fruits, raisins, almonds, dates, boiled milk, lassi, and fresh cheeses.

Rajasic foods encourage action; they create "karma." Meats are rajasic, as are foods that are overly salty, spicy, sour, or sharp.

Tamasic foods are counter evolutionary. They lead to cloudy thinking and keep you stuck where you are. Examples include leftovers, processed food, fast food, junk food, microwaved food, mushrooms, and many foods that grow in the ground (such as potatoes, and peanuts). Note that onions and garlic are both tamasic foods and should not be used in excess (asafetida is a good substitute).

It is important to include all 3 types of foods in the diet, but one should favor sattvic foods as much as possible, while maintaining limits on the intake of rajasic and tamasic foods.

Eat In A Settled Environment

We must set aside enough time to sit down and have a decent lunch every day. This is going to take at minimum 20 to 30 minutes. When we eat, we eat. That's it. We don't eat and read. We don't eat and watch TV. We don't eat and read our e-mails. We don't eat while we're driving. We try not to eat during meetings. When we eat, we simply sit there quietly and eat. Light and pleasant conversation is okay, but no yelling or arguing. When we eat, we should be sitting, not standing. We commonly see people at dinner parties eating while standing but this should be avoided. Have a seat, relax, and enjoy your food.

Fresh Is Best

Favor fresh food. When we are talking about fruits and vegetables, that's the produce section of the store, not the canned or the frozen food section. We will all eat canned and frozen sometimes, but it shouldn't be the habit. As a general rule, foods that are processed, foods that are packaged, and foods with lots of additives are all less healthy in comparison with good, old-fashioned, fresh food.

In ayurveda, we reduce or avoid leftovers. This of course means that someone needs to cook every day; you, someone you know, someone you hire, or some combination of the above. We'll all eat leftovers sometimes, but it shouldn't be the habit.

> How does this work in the real world? Chapter Three provides multiple recipe options that can be cooked overnight in your slow cooker then carried with you to work in a thermos for a delicious, fresh, home cooked hot lunch! You can then reheat for dinner, but try not to hold things overnight.

If you forget to start your slow cooker meal the night before, another thing you can try is the "thermos-cooked lunch" (see recipe for Thermos-Cooked Lunch). Using this technique, you get your bean and grain started first thing in the morning, then place the partially cooked meal in a wide-mouth thermos. The food continues cooking in the thermos during the course of the morning, and is fresh and ready by lunch.

Why is eating fresh so important? When food lies around for too long, it begins to oxidize. Let's suppose you make a casserole on a Sunday, and you eat half of it. The remainder gets shoved into the refrigerator. The casserole then somehow works its way to the rear corner of your refrigerator. Half a year later, you are cleaning the fridge, and there you find it! Would you eat it? Of course not, it's disgusting. That process of deterioration begins right away. Of course, 2 days in the refrigerator is different from 6 months, but as a general rule you want to cook and eat your food the same day.

In this context, we also emphasize that people should as much as possible *avoid using the microwave oven*. In ayurveda, we maintain that the microwave oven has an inauspicious influence on food. Speed of cooking is important. Slow cooking brings out the flavor and makes the food more digestible. The microwave, in contrast, causes the molecules in the food to vibrate at an extremely rapid rate, which has a vata aggravating effect on the food. In addition, use of the microwave encourages the consumption of leftovers, processed foods, and frozen foods. From an ayurvedic perspective, we consider all microwaved foods to be tamasic. The way you cook your food will effect your physiology and consciousness. Slow-cooked food will nourish the physiology; microwaving will do the opposite.

THERMOS-COOKED LUNCH

We advise using a vacuum-sealed, wide-mouth stainless steel or glass-core thermos. The stainless steel thermos is best because it won't break like the glass ones sometimes do. The vacuum seal is important, because a vacuum-sealed thermos continues to cook the food more efficiently.

Ingredients:

1 T of ghee or olive oil
Whole or ground spices to taste (salt, pepper, cumin, ginger, turmeric, etc.)
¼ cup yellow split mung beans
½ cup basmati rice
1½ cups of fresh vegetables, cut into small pieces to fit into a thermos (slower-cooking vegetables like carrots, celery, kale, green beans, and sweet potatoes work best because they won't overcook)
2 cups water

Directions:

1. Clean the rice and dahl.
2. Saute the spices in the ghee for a few minutes on low-medium heat. Add the mung dal, rice, and chopped vegetables.
3. Pour the water over the mixture, bring to a boil, and cook 5-10 minutes.
4. While still boiling, pour the mixture into a 1 quart or 1 liter thermos. You may need to ladle or spoon it in, but work quickly so that it doesn't cool down.
5. Seal the thermos right away and leave it closed for about 4 hours.
6. The meal will cook in the thermos and be ready to eat after 4 hours!

The science on this is controversial; however, several lines of experimental evidence support the recommendation that people avoid using microwave ovens. For one, microwave ovens have the potential to leak radiation, which can theoretically increase the risk of cancer, birth defects, and other medical problems.[28] Second, microwaving has been found to have a detrimental effect on human breast milk.[29] Researchers discovered that microwaving breast milk at high temperatures (72 to 98 degrees Centigrade) caused a marked decrease in activity of anti-infective factors. The growth of *Escherichia* coli (E coli) bacteria in the microwaved milk was 18 times higher than in that of control human milk. Microwaving food can alter the chemical structure of the nutrients. One study[30] showed that microwaves cause a higher degree of "protein unfolding" than conventional heating. Finally, microwaving foods can adversely impact their nutritional value. For example, investigators have found that microwaving broccoli causes a 97% reduction in beneficial antioxidants, compared with steaming, which has minimal effect.[31] Another study[32] likewise showed that steaming broccoli was superior to microwaving, as well as to other common domestic cooking methods, in terms of retention of nutrients.

Is It Important To Buy Organic Products?

We advise patients to choose organic produce and products as much as possible. Sometimes this may not be feasible economically, but when possible, it is best to buy and eat organic foods. As a general rule, this may be more important for products that do not require peeling vs those that do: One might tolerate conventionally grown (not organic) oranges and bananas, but choose organic berries or cherries.

The Environmental Work Group maintains an inventory of conventionally grown produce with the highest concentration of contaminants.[33] These are products that would be most important to purchase organic. The 2018 "dirty dozen" among conventionally grown produce, in descending order (worst is first) include strawberries, spinach, nectarines, apples, grapes, peaches, cherries, pears, tomatoes, celery, potatoes, and sweet bell peppers.

Is It Okay To Consume Beer Or Wine? How About Coffee?

In ayurveda, we maintain that alcohol is a toxin, tolerable in small amounts. It is okay to have a single glass of wine or bottle of beer with your meal, but as always, the drink should be room temperature, not cold. On the other hand, hard alcohol should be completely avoided.

Caffeine is a stimulant that imbalances both vata and pitta doshas, but can balance kapha. If a patient has a kapha constitution, a few cups of coffee during the course of the day could be appropriate. For the rest of us, coffee and other caffeinated beverages should be avoided or reduced. A single cup of coffee in the morning is generally no big deal, especially during cold, wet weather.

Honey: The Exception To The Rule

We have to this point done a considerable amount of ranting and raving about cooking everything. The rule in ayurveda is cook your food. Every rule, of course, has an exception. Fresh fruit has been cooked by the sun, so you don't have to cook it. However you can cook fresh fruit if you like. Harder fruits, such as apples or pears are wonderful when cooked, but you don't have to cook them, unless you want to. There is one important exception to the "cook your food" rule, and that is honey. Honey is an ideal sweetener, raw.

According to ayurveda, cooked honey is toxic. There is something about cooking honey that generates a lot of ama. If you take honey that has been heated, or pasteurized, and feed it to bees, it will kill the bees. So, whereas raw honey is an ideal sweetener, people should avoid cooked honey.

This means that when you purchase honey at the store, make sure it says "raw" on the label. When you purchase baked goods, look on the label. If there is honey cooked into it, don't buy it. If you go to the bread section of most health food stores, and you look at the labels, the great majority of the breads on the shelves have honey cooked into them. Leave these on the shelves, and buy another instead. Cooking with other sweeteners, such as cane sugar, fruit juice, or molasses, is fine; just don't cook with honey.

You can put honey in your tea once the tea is sufficiently cooled down such that you can place and hold your finger in the tea (about 115 degrees Fahrenheit). You can add honey to a warm drink, but not to a boiling hot drink.

From the standpoint of modern science, the reason for the deleterious effects of cooked honey may be related to the chemical hydroxymethyl furfuraldehyde (HMF). Scientists who have studied the nutritional composition of honey have reported a significant rise in HMF in honey samples that have been heated to 60° C (140° F) and 140° C (284° F).[34] Concerns have been raised about HMF as a potential carcinogen.[35]

SUMMARY POINTS: GUIDELINES TO PROPER DIGESTION

Have your main meal at lunch. Dinner should be lighter.

Snacking is okay, but no grazing. After eating, allow three hours to digest your food before you eat again. Avoid snacking at night.

No cold beverages—even water. Room temperature beverages are fine, and warm drinks are most beneficial.

Food should be cooked and consumed warm, or at least room temperature. Fresh fruit need not be cooked, but raw vegetables and other raw foods should be reduced or avoided.

The ideal diet is a lactovegetarian diet (a vegetarian diet that includes dairy products).

Cold milk should be avoided. Milk should be boiled and consumed hot. Milk should be combined with sweet-tasting foods only.

Fresh cheeses are much better than aged cheeses.

Lassi, a yogurt drink, is easy to digest and provides probiotic support.

Clarified butter, ghee, is an excellent oil for cooking.

Eat in a settled environment.

Fresh is best!

Raw honey is an ideal sweetener. Avoid cooked honey.

CHAPTER FIVE

SHOW ME THE MENU!

Menus specifically tailored to individual constitutional types.

The guidelines to proper digestion outlined in the previous chapters apply to most everyone. In addition to these, on the basis of which dosha you need to balance, we will recommend that specific people favor or avoid specific foods. On the following pages you will find 3 sample diets: a vata-balancing diet, a pitta-balancing diet, and a kapha-balancing diet. Each diet lists foods that one should favor, or avoid, to balance that particular dosha. The short answer is, you can look at your questionnaire score, look at the score that was highest, turn to the corresponding diet, and follow it. Another good approach for some people is to eat according to the season. That is to say, favor a pitta-balancing diet when the weather is hot, a vata-blancing diet when the weather is cold and windy, and a kapha-balancing diet when the weather is cold and wet. Guidance from a physician or dietician, as well as trial and error, can provide further help with specifying food selections. You can review the diets on the following pages, or in other books, or on the Internet, and easily find long lists of foods that balance or imbalance a particular dosha. We will first present a chart describing the rationale for determining the impact that a particular food may have on a particular dosha. We can care for our health more effectively by understanding the rationale behind each of the diets above and beyond simply memorizing a long list of foods to favor or avoid.

An individual food will affect a particular dosha as a function of the *tastes* and the *qualities* of that food. There are 3 doshas, as already reviewed, and there are 6 tastes. The 6 tastes are sweet, sour, salty, bitter, pungent (indicating hot and spicy, like chili peppers), and astringent. Astringent foods make your mouth pucker up a little bit, like beans or pomegranates. An unripe persimmon exemplifies an extremely astringent food.

> The tastes are six. They are sweet, sour, saline, pungent, bitter and astringent. Properly used, they nourish the body. Improperly used (excess or deficient), they verily lead to the provocation of the Dosha. The Dosha are three: Vata, Pitta and Kapha. When they are in their normal state, they are beneficial to the body. When, however, they become disorganized, verily they afflict the body with diseases of diverse kinds.
>
> — Charaka Samhita, 3.1.3-4

	TASTES						QUALITIES					
DOSHA	SWEET	SOUR	SALTY	BITTER	PUNGENT	ASTRINGENT	WARM	COOL	DRY	OILY	HEAVY	LIGHT
VATTA	▼	▼	▼	△	△	△	▼	△	△	▼	▼	△
PITTA	▼	△	△	▼	△	▼	△	▼	△	▼	▼	△
KAPHA	△	△	△	▼	▼	▼	▼	△	▼	△	△	▼

Tastes and food qualities as they impact the doshas. A downward arrow indicates that the taste or quality reduces, or helps to balance, that dosha.

In addition to the 6 tastes, there are 6 qualities of foods. Foods can be either heating or cooling; salsa is heating, cucumbers are cooling. Foods can be either heavy or light. Foods can be either oily or dry.

For vata dosha, sweet, sour, and salty tastes reduce the influence of or balance vata dosha. If you look at the vata-balancing diet, you find lots of sweet, sour, and salty tasting foods on the menu, with relatively little in the way of bitter, pungent, or astringent tastes. Vata is cold, so you need heating foods to balance it. Vata is light, so you need heavy foods to balance it. Vata is dry, so you need oily foods to balance it. In sum then, the vata-balancing diet consists primarily of sweet, sour, salty, heating, heavy, oily foods, while reducing or avoiding bitter, pungent, astringent, cooling, light, and dry foods. Keep in mind that a classic vata diet might make you gain a little weight. If you are like most people in North America, you probably are not eager to gain weight. In that case, the vata diet can still be appropriate, but be sure to watch the amount of heavy, oily foods.

For kapha, bitter, pungent, and astringent tasting foods reduce the influence of, or balance, kapha dosha. Thus the kapha-balancing diet consists primarily of bitter, pungent, and astringent tasting foods, while reducing or avoiding sweet, sour and salty tastes. This is the best diet for weight loss, because it is the lightest of the diets. The kapha-balancing diet is also helpful in the setting of respiratory congestion. If you have a sinus infection, or if your child or grandchild has problems with colds, middle ear infections, or asthma, *do* eat foods that are bitter, pungent, astringent, heating, light, and dry. At the same time, *do not eat* foods that are sweet, sour, salty, cooling, heavy, or oily. In other words, if you have a sinus infection, don't eat ice cream! This may seem obvious, but it is surprising how many people, including many physicians, don't get it. In the same way, if your child or grandchild is having problems with asthma, middle ear infections, etc., don't give him or her cold juice or cold milk out of the refrigerator. These drinks are both cold and sweet. They will aggravate kapha, i.e., stimulate mucus production, and exacerbate the problem. In fact, if the child has been consuming lots of cold milk, cold juice, and/or cold soft drinks, this could even be the primary cause of the problem. Favoring flatbreads, such as pita bread, chapatis, and tortillas, while reducing or eliminating puffy breads, will also help correct kapha imbalance. In either case, always toast the bread. Flatbreads are lighter and easier to digest than leavened breads, especially untoasted leavened breads.

Finally, to balance pitta dosha, favor foods that are sweet, bitter, astringent, cooling, and moderate in terms of heaviness and oil. With the pitta-balancing diet, we are careful to reduce or avoid sour, salty, pungent, and heating foods.

Note that all of the food items in the diets that follow are lactovegetarian choices: no beef, no poultry, no fish, no eggs. As mentioned previously, a lactovegetarian diet is favored, but not required. If you do eat meat, we recommend you do so at lunchtime. Poultry (chicken) is preferred, then fish, with red meats last. Of the red meats, favor lamb over beef and pork.

The Use Of Spices Is Very Important!

Each of the diets includes a recipe for a convenient dosha-specific spice mix, as well as a list of spices that are favorable for balancing that dosha. Ayurveda emphasizes the importance of cooking with plenty of spices on a daily basis. These spices help to ignite agni and to properly digest and assimilate the food. The spices also provide a range of additional health benefits, including modulation of detoxification enzymes, stimulation of the immune system, and reduction of inflammation. Many spices also possess antioxidant, antibacterial, and antiviral properties.[36] Finally, selecting and using the proper spices also goes a long way toward correcting and preventing imbalances of the relevant dosha.

VATA-PACIFYING DIET

SPICE MIX FOR BALANCING VATA DOSHA

Ingredients:
8 tsp ground cumin
8 tsp ground fennel
2 tsp ground coriander
2 tsp ground turmeric
1 tsp ground ginger
¼ tsp ground cinnamon

Directions:
Mix these spices and keep the mix in a shaker to use with meals.

General Approach

Favor foods that are sweet, sour, salty, heavy, oily, and heating, while reducing or avoiding foods that are bitter, pungent, astringent, light, dry, and cooling. It is very important to eat fresh food and to eat on a regular routine.

GRAINS

Favor: wheat, rice.

Reduce: barley, corn, millet, buckwheat, rye.

LEGUMES

Favor: yellow split mung beans, garbanzos, red lentils, tofu.

Reduce: all other beans.

NUTS

Favor: almost all nuts are generally good.

Reduce: peanuts.

VEGETABLES

Favor: eggplant (peeled), zucchini, cucumber, asparagus, artichoke, tomato (peeled), celery, carrots, beets, and spinach. Just about all vegetables are good, but vegetables must be cooked, generally with a little bit of ghee or other oil.

Reduce: raw vegetables.

DAIRY PRODUCTS

Favor: whole or low-fat cow's milk, goat milk, buttermilk, lassi, ghee (clarified butter), cream cheese, cottage cheese, panir, other fresh cheeses

Reduce: ice cream.

SWEETENERS

Favor: most healthy sweeteners are okay, including cane sugar, brown sugar, molasses, and raw honey.

Reduce: processed sugars, high-fructose corn syrup.

OILS

Favor: most oils are good for reducing vata.

Reduce: coconut oil (because of its cooling properties).

SPICES & CONDIMENTS

Favor: cumin, ginger, fenugreek, hing (asafetida), mustard seed, black pepper, cinnamon, cardamom, anise, fennel, cloves, salt, lemon juice, tamarind, basil, clove, mint, nutmeg, bay leaf, fenugreek, turmeric, paprika.

Reduce: red pepper and chili.

FRUITS

Favor: sweet, sour, heavy, and ripe fruits are ideal. Grapes, papayas, pineapples, bananas, avocados, cherries, peaches, melons, figs, plums, mangoes, papayas, pineapples, oranges, and fresh apricots are good. Raisins are good but should first be soaked overnight in warm water.

Reduce: dried fruits (unless soaked overnight in water just to cover), apples, cranberries.

PITTA-PACIFYING DIET

SPICE MIX FOR BALANCING PITTA DOSHA

Directions:

Mix these spices and keep in a shaker to use with meals.

Ingredients:

10 tsp ground fennel
4 tsp ground coriander
2 tsp ground turmeric

General Approach

Favor foods that are sweet, bitter, astringent, cooling, and moderate in terms of oil. Avoid sour, salty, pungent, hot, spicy foods. Stay away from vinegar and acidic foods.

GRAINS

Favor: wheat, rice, barley, oats.

Reduce: corn, millet, rye, buckwheat.

LEGUMES

Favor: yellow split mung beans, adzuki beans, navy beans, garbanzos, lentils, tofu.

Reduce: other beans.

VEGETABLES

Favor: asparagus, artichokes, yellow squash, zucchini, okra, spinach (in small amounts), cauliflower, broccoli, cabbage, green beans, celery, sweet potatoes, peas, bell pepper, sprouts, lettuce, cucumber, tender eggplant, leafy greens.

Reduce: tomatoes, tomato sauce, radish, onions.

DAIRY

Favor: milk, butter, ghee (clarified butter), sweet lassi, cream, cream cheese, panir (homemade cheese from milk).

Reduce: yogurt, aged or salty cheese, salty butter, sour cream.

SWEETENERS

Favor: cane sugar, raw honey (but not in excess), date sugar.

Reduce: molasses, brown sugar.

OILS

Favor: olive, sunflower, ghee, coconut.

Reduce: almond, corn, safflower, sesame, canola.

NUTS & SEEDS

Favor: sunflower and pumpkin seeds, blanched almonds.

Reduce: other nuts and seeds.

SPICES

Favor: coriander, cilantro, cumin, fresh ginger root (in small amounts), turmeric, saffron, fennel, cinnamon, cardamom, black pepper (in small amounts), lemon juice, thyme, basil, oregano, marjoram (in small amounts).

Reduce: chile pepper, cayenne, garlic, mustard seed, cloves, celery seed, fenugreek, salt.

FRUITS

Favor: sweet grapes, avocado, mango, coconut, melons, kiwi, sweet oranges, sweet plums, papaya, sweet pineapple, persimmon, pomegranate, cherries.

Reduce: grapefruit, olives, sour orange, peach, sour grapes, sour pineapple, berries, cranberries, prunes.

KAPHA-PACIFYING DIET

SPICE MIX FOR BALANCING KAPHA DOSHA

Directions:

Mix these spices and keep the mixture in a shaker to use with meals.

Ingredients:

6 tsp ground coriander
6 tsp ground cumin
3 tsp ground turmeric
2 tsp ground fenugreek (if this is hard to find, you can grind fenugreek seeds in your blender)
¼ tsp ground ginger
¼ tsp ground black pepper

General Approach

Favor bitter, pungent, and astringent tastes, while avoiding sweet, sour, and salty tastes. Favor light, heating, dry foods while reducing heavy, cold, and oily foods. Avoid sugar, sweets, and frozen desserts.

GRAINS

Favor: barley, millet, corn, buckwheat, rye (All grains should ideally be a minimum of 1 year old).

Reduce: wheat and rice.

LEGUMES

Favor: almost all beans are appropriate.

Reduce: tofu.

VEGETABLES

Favor: green leafy vegetables, asparagus, carrots, beets, potatoes, tomatoes, artichoke, celery, white pumpkin, cabbage, cauliflower, peas, bell pepper, sprouts, tender eggplant, tender radish.

Reduce: sweet potatoes, cucumbers, zucchini.

DAIRY

Favor: low fat or skim milk (boiled and served hot), small amounts of ghee, lassi.

Reduce: yogurt, cream, butter, whole milk and ghee in large quantities.

SWEETENERS

Favor: raw honey.

Reduce: all other sweeteners.

OILS

Favor: very small amounts of ghee, mustard, almond, and sesame oil, (all used sparingly).

Reduce: all oils in general.

NUTS & SEEDS

Favor: sunflower and pumpkin seeds.

Reduce: nuts in general.

SPICES

Favor: almost all spices, especially ginger, black pepper, turmeric, cinnamon, mustard seed, cloves, mint, paprika, basil, fenugreek.

Reduce: salt.

FRUITS

Favor: grapes (red), peaches, apples, pears, raisins, persimmon, dried figs, papaya, guava, pomegranate, cranberries.

Reduce: avocado, banana, coconut, pineapple, oranges, melons, plums, prunes, grapes (green), oranges, mango, apricots, fresh figs, dates, melons.

Jerusalem Spice Shop

(oil on canvas)

Welcome to the world of spices, where warm colors, enticing aromas, and pungent tastes fire the digestion! Various spices glow in their jars, or beckon from huge peaked piles. The woman in the spice shop radiates confidence because she possesses the knowledge of the properties of these spices. A savvy shopper, she can confidently select precisely those spices that will both best flavor the food, and optimally promote ideal digestion and balanced health for her family.

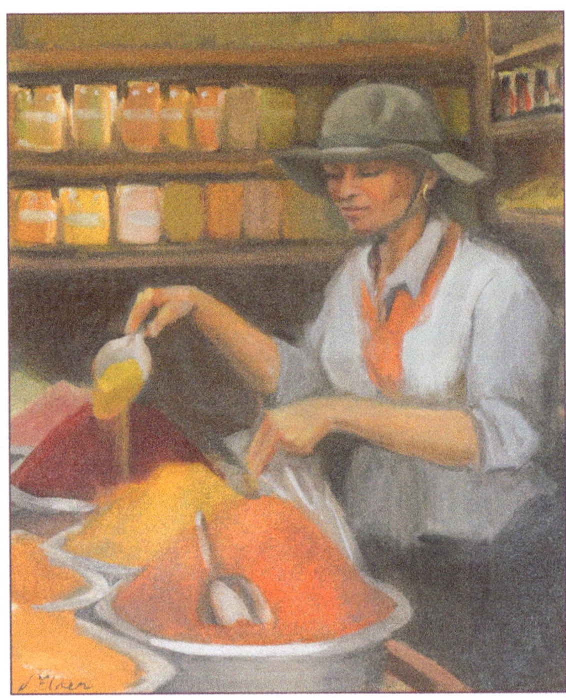

CHAPTER SIX

EARLY TO BED, EARLY TO RISE, EXERCISE IN THE MORNING, AND HAVE A DECENT LUNCH

How and why to optimize your daily routine.

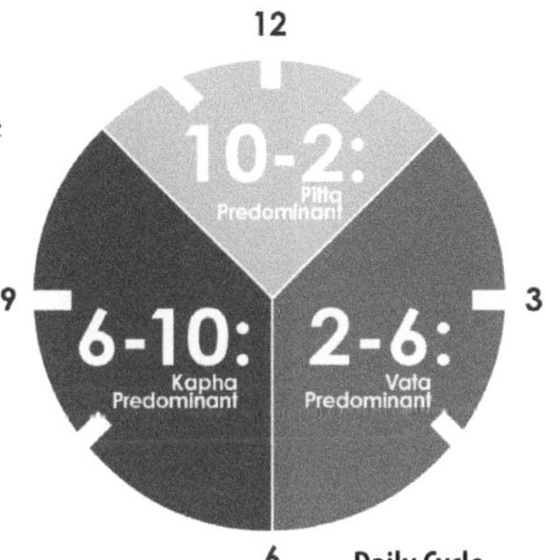

Daily Cycle of the Doshas

The next topic will be daily routine and exercise. You see in the figure: Daily Cycle of The Doshas, a clock describing the daily cycle of the doshas. Recall from Chapter One that there is a seasonal cycle of the doshas: Summer is pitta season, winter is vata season, and spring is kapha season. There is likewise a lifetime cycle of the doshas: Youth is the kapha season of life, midlife is the pitta season of life, and the last part of life is the vata season of life. In the same way, there is a daily cycle of the doshas.

Ten a.m. to 2 p.m. is the pitta period of the day. As the sun is rising to its highest point in the sky, pitta dosha increases in everyone. During this period, the qualities of pitta dosha predominate in nature and the environment. Two p.m. to 6 p.m. is the vata period of the day, and 6 p.m. to 10 p.m. is the kapha period of the evening. The cycle then resumes; 10 p.m. to 2 a.m. is the pitta period of the night, 2 a.m. to 6 a.m. is the vata period of the early morning, and 6 a.m. to 10 a.m. is the kapha period of the morning. Thus we have four-hour blocks of time, times 3 doshas makes 12 hours, repeated twice makes 24 hours. At any given moment, day or night, we are in one of these periods.

With this framework in mind, and reflecting back on what we learned about the doshas in Chapter One, we can now construct our ideal daily routine. If you would like this rhythm, this natural daily cycle of the doshas, to be working in your favor rather than against you, what should your daily routine look like? How do we structure our daily routine to harness support of nature in our daily activities? Stated another way, what should you do when, each day, to assure that as you go through your day, and life, you are paddling your canoe with the current as opposed to upstream?

We'll start at the beginning of the day. Six a.m. to 10 a.m. is the kapha period of the morning. Kapha is the heavy, physical dosha. What do you want to make sure you do every day before this period starts? Wake up! *Out of bed by 6 a.m. every day.* That experience of waking up dull and groggy at 8 a.m. or even 9 a.m. is from sleeping into the kapha period of the day. Vata, in contrast, is light and energetic. Assuming we got to bed on time the night before, waking up during the vata period of the morning is ideal: The lightness and energy of vata dosha will stick with you throughout the day.

> **They have given another principle with regard to physical well-being:**
> **As long as one exercises, exerts himself greatly, does not eat to the point of satiation and has loose bowels, he will not suffer sickness and he will grow in strength.**
> **[This applies] even if he eats harmful foods.**
> — Maimonides, **Mishneh Torah,** Hilchot De'ot 4:14.

The best time to exercise is between 6 a.m. and 10 a.m., during the kapha period of the morning. (see Sidebar: Should You Eat Before Exercising?) The second-best time to exercise is between 6 p.m. and 10 p.m., during the kapha period of the evening. The prescription, then, is nothing new; wake up early and get some exercise! The heavy physical qualities of kapha render this the most natural time for physical activity. In ayurveda we emphasize that exercise should help remove stress from, not create stress for, the physiology. There is no need to train for a decathlon, unless you want to. A brisk walk counts as exercise and is appropriate and healthy for the great majority of people. If you are interested in doing something more intense, for example running 6 miles, you are much less likely to injure yourself if you do so during the kapha period, as opposed to other times of the day.

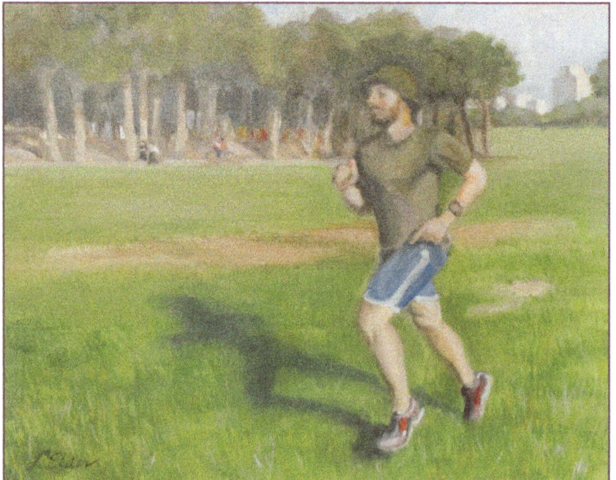

Morning Run
(oil on canvas)

Early morning presents the best time for exercise. The painting depicts a runner, walkers, and a cyclist enjoying a clear autumn morning at Saker Park in Jerusalem. Making a routine of exercising most days, and sticking with it, prevents disease, promotes vitality, and is essential for long-term health.

SHOULD YOU EAT BEFORE EXERCISING?

If you are working out early in the morning as recommended, should you eat first? Results from one interesting study[37] help lend some insight. In this experiment, the research team recruited 27 healthy male volunteers and fed them a high-calorie, high-fat diet for 6 weeks. The investigators divided the participants into 3 groups. The first group consumed the high-calorie diet and participated in a rigorous exercise program in the morning before eating. The second group participated in the same exercise program, but consumed a carbohydrate-rich breakfast 90 minutes before exercise. They also had a carbohydrate-enriched drink during exercise. The third group consumed the high-calorie diet but did not participate in any exercise program. The investigators found that only those in the first group who exercised before eating showed improvements in glucose tolerance and insulin sensitivity. This group also demonstrated beneficial metabolic adaptations in muscle cells that can help improve insulin sensitivity.

Whether or not you should eat in the morning before exercising will depend upon a variety of factors, including your body type, digestion, food selection, exercise intensity, and so on. The results of this study suggest that all else equal, it may be preferable to exercise first thing in the morning *before* having a big breakfast.

We can also recommend specific types of exercise, geared toward specific types of people. Vata types should favor calming types of exercise, such as walking or yoga, while kapha types should favor more stimulating exercise, such as jogging or racquetball. Pitta types can do most any exercise, but should avoid intense competition.

Out of bed early, then between 6 a.m. and 10 a.m. in the morning, during the kapha period, we exercise. *Ten a.m. to 2 p.m.* is the pitta period of the day, with the sun rising to its highest point in the sky. This will be the ideal time for doing what? As we've said multiple times, *eating your biggest meal!* Then, 2 p.m. to 6 p.m. is the vata period of the afternoon. This is the proper time for mental activity.

Some people report feeling drowsy after lunch, and because of this they have difficulty with mental concentration in the afternoon. In truth, if we eat a proper lunch, the main meal should make us feel *more* light and clear for the afternoon's work. Drowsiness after lunch signals ama production, caused by weak digestion, unwholesome food, eating too fast, eating too much, or some combination of the above.

Now the cycle resumes. Six p.m. to 10 p.m. is the kapha period of the evening. What do we want to be sure to do before this period ends? Do what by 10 p.m.? Get to bed! You don't have to be asleep by 10 p.m., but *in bed, lights out, television off, by 10 p.m.!* We want our sleep to be heavy. Turn the lights out and lie down by 10 p.m., and the heavy quality of kapha will spill over into your sleep. If, however, we make the mistake of staying up too late, 10 p.m. to 2 a.m. is the pitta time of night. Pitta is intense, we get a second wind, and then it's even harder to fall asleep. We've all had that experience. In addition, there's an even better reason to get to bed by 10 p.m. We said that pitta governs digestion and metabolism. During the pitta time of day, between 10 a.m. and 2 p.m., we eat and digest our biggest meal. During the pitta time of night, between 10 p.m. and 2 a.m., we metabolize and process the day's wastes. This is when the clean-up crew comes in. It is very important to be in bed by 10 p.m., then, so the body can properly cleanse itself. If we are habitually awake and busy during this nighttime pitta period, the natural cleansing processes are inhibited, and ama starts to accumulate, thus setting the stage for potential disease or illness. This is why it is so critically important for your long-term health to get to bed on a regular basis by 10 p.m.

The table below outlines the essentials of the ayurvedic daily routine:

Daily routine		
Time	**Predominant Dosha**	**Activity**
2 a.m. - 6 a.m.	Vata	Wake up
6 a.m. - 10 a.m.	Kapha	Exercise
10 a.m. - 2 p.m.	Pitta	Eat
2 p.m. - 6 p.m.	Vata	Mental activity
6 p.m. - 10 p.m.	Kapha	Exercise and go to bed
10 p.m. - 2 a.m.	Pitta	Sleep

To summarize this daily routine, then, in the simplest possible terms: Early to bed, early to rise, get some exercise in the morning, and have a decent lunch. Next day: Early to bed, early to rise, get some exercise in the morning, and have a decent lunch. Next day: Early to bed, early to rise, get some exercise in the morning, and have a decent lunch. There you have it, the *picture of health*. If everyone followed this simple routine, there would be far fewer sick people, and our primary care clinics would have many more open appointments!

What if you work a swing shift? Let's say you work from 2 p.m. until 10 p.m., 5 days a week. What then? This schedule may not be ideal, but we can manage with it. Have your main meal at midday before going to work, then a light dinner during your break at work, but be sure not to munch on junk food on the job. When you get home at night, don't eat. Instead, get to bed as soon as you can. Not perfect, but close enough.

What if you are working a graveyard shift? This is not sustainable, and we encourage our patients to switch off of the graveyard shift whenever feasible. Data suggest that people who work graveyard shifts suffer from a range of related health problems,[38] including increased risk of breast cancer and cardiovascular death.[39]

Is it okay to nap during the day? Napping is fine if you are ill, if you are elderly, or if the weather is extremely hot. Beyond these situations, as a general principle, you should avoid daytime napping.

Some patients will object, "I'm not a morning person," or "I'm just a night person," or something to this effect. We should not view chronically staying up too late, or oversleeping in the morning, as some neutral innate personality characteristic, but rather as a bad habit. Imagine going into your backyard in the middle of the day to do some gardening, and seeing a bat flying around in broad daylight. You pull out your phone to call the health department, and the bat objects, "No worry, I'm a day bat." Of course there is no such thing as a day bat. Bats work at night, and sleep during the day. Likewise for raccoons. People, in contrast, are not nocturnal creatures. We work by day, and sleep by night.

PART II.
GENERALLY SPEAKING

*An overview of approaches
we recommend to most patients,
and a review of contemporary topics
in the field of complementary
and integrative medicine*

CHAPTER SEVEN

MIND YOUR BODY

Understand the different types of mind-body techniques, and which may be best for you.

In a landmark article in 1970, Dr. Keith Wallace published the results of a study evaluating whether meditation practice could induce measurable changes in the physiology.[40] He recruited study participants and assessed their physiologic patterns before, during, and after Transcendental Meditation (TM) practice. Dr. Wallace documented that, during TM, subjects' oxygen consumption and heart rate decreased, and skin resistance increased. In addition, he reported specific changes in the electroencephalogram (EEG or brain wave) patterns. The findings were of high importance. Many people had thought of meditation as just some type of counterculture mood-making phenomenon. Not so. The study showed that a simple mental stress reduction technique could bring about measurable changes in the practitioner's physiology. In other words, a person can achieve relaxation of the body through a structured approach to relaxing the mind! By extension, if the mind can change the body in measurable ways, then meditation techniques may not be just for those who want a tool to help relax. Potentially, meditation can be used to prevent, or treat, not only mental but also physical health problems.

In the decades since, meditation techniques have indeed been shown effective in the management of a number of chronic medical conditions. Mind and body are of course connected, so this should come as no surprise. Even so, these techniques remain underutilized in the setting of chronic disease management. Why institute chronic drug therapy, with all the associated cost, potential inconvenience, and side effects, if a self-help mind-body approach such as meditation can work just as well or better? Why rely on a physician, or complementary medicine practitioner, to provide you with some sort of treatment, if instruction in a simple meditation technique can empower you to heal yourself?

Meditation techniques involve much more than just randomly sitting there with your eyes closed. We should think of the word "science" as denoting any branch or department of systematized knowledge considered as a distinct field of investigation or object of study. That "science" connotes empiricism is not an a priori truth but rather a provincialism of our culture.[41] An authentic meditation technique, then, can be properly understood as a scientific pursuit, being a tool for systematic study of mind, being, consciousness, and the self.

Research into Consciousness
(oil on canvas)
The soft light and tender colors in this painting communicate something of the experience of deep meditation.

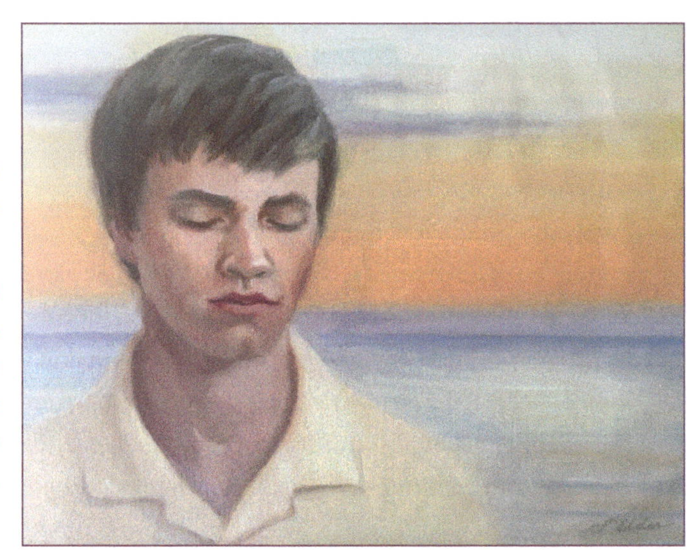

There is not just one type of meditation. Rather, meditation techniques come in many different types, and it is important to understand that they are not necessarily interchangeable. The physiologic imprint and specific clinical benefit of meditation will vary on the basis of the type of meditation practiced. To take an analogy, we may determine that a patient has an infection and needs an antibiotic. But which antibiotic? Many antibiotics are available and clearly they are not all exactly alike. The physician decides which antibiotic to recommend on the basis of the source of the infection, the types of germs that are likely to be involved, and a host of other factors. In the same way, a range of different meditation techniques are available, serving a range of purposes and producing a variety of effects. Thus it may not be so useful to place all types of meditation approaches under one umbrella. Rather, one should understand which types of techniques are available, what they have in common, and how they differ. Ultimately, both physicians and patients should gain a sense for the pros and cons of the various techniques, and which may be most suitable for a particular medical indication or type of person.

The job of classifying meditation techniques is a difficult one owing to a number of factors. Many techniques are available, emanating from different cultures, traditions, and historic eras. Any particular practice may fall into more than one category, under different circumstances, or perhaps even during the same meditation session. For these and other reasons, achieving a universally applicable classification scheme can be difficult.

Dr. Fred Travis, in a paper published in *Consciousness and Cognition,* proposed categorizing meditation practices into 3 types,[42] on the basis of their purpose, practice, and neurophysiologic imprint. The 3 types of meditation are focused-attention, open monitoring, and automatic self-transcending techniques.

Focused-attention techniques include those approaches that involve focusing the mind on a particular object or emotion, such as a stick of burning incense. The meditator focuses attention entirely on this one thing. Practicing such techniques can then serve to improve one's ability to focus attention during activity. This would be good training for tasks such as studying for an examination. In focused-attention meditation, the brain is working hard. Using an EEG to measure the electrical activity of the brain during focused-attention meditation, the pattern shows a type of electrical waves called gamma waves, at a rate of 20Hz to 50Hz. Examples of focused-attention meditation include Zen meditation, compassion meditation, qigong, and diamond way Buddhism.

Open-monitoring techniques involve observing, or shifting attention toward or being mindful of, one's breath or thoughts. Thoughts pass through the mind, and the meditator is training herself or himself to dispassionately observe them. Or, the meditator mentally attends to the movement of the breath, and dispassionately observes. The intended outcome is to cultivate a nonjudgmental attitude toward experience. During open-monitoring meditation, the mind is watching, or observing, itself, and the associated EEG pattern shows theta2 waves, at a rate of 6 Hz to 8 Hz. This is the pattern you see when the mind is turned within and is observing mental processes. Examples include Mindfulness meditation, Za Zen, and Kriya Yoga.

The third type of meditation, automatic self-transcending techniques, involves transcending the steps of meditation practice. The experience in this case is to take the mind to its inner source of silence and alertness. The practitioner transcends his or her own thoughts and activity, usually through the use of a mantra (repetition of a silent word without meaning). During practice of automatic self-transcending techniques, with the attention simply awake and turned within, the EEG pattern shows alpha 1 waves at 8 Hz to 10 Hz, with this alpha 1 pattern seen throughout the entire brain. Examples include TM, and long-term qigong practice.

In summary, people use focused-attention and open-monitoring techniques to construct mental tools during meditation to be used after the meditation. These techniques teach how to use the mind in a specific way, to better take care of a particular situation or task. In the case of focused-attention, one is training in the skill of maintaining the mind's focus. In the case of open-monitoring techniques, one is cultivating a nonjudgmental attitude toward experience. In the case of automatic self-transcending techniques, the aim is an overall change in the mental state. In this type of meditation, the goal is not to train the practitioner how to use the mind in a certain way, but rather to clarify and enhance the overall function of the mind.

Of the many available techniques, two in particular are both popular in North America, and have been the focus of considerable scientific scrutiny. These are TM and Mindfulness-Based Stress Reduction (MBSR).

TM is an example of an automatic self-transcending technique. TM can be thought of as a simple mental technique for managing stress. TM was introduced to the west by Maharishi Mahesh Yogi in the late 1950s, and is derived from the Vedic tradition. Some people think that meditation sounds like a difficult chore but it turns out that TM is extremely easy to do. For the purposes of scientific assessment and dissemination, important advantages of the TM program include a standardized and reproducible instruction format, a thorough certification program for instructors, and widespread availability of instructors in essentially all population centers in North America. TM is performed twice daily for 15-20 minutes while sitting quietly with eyes closed in a comfortable position. This meditation technique allows the mind to experience finer levels of the thinking process and to achieve a state of deep relaxation. TM practice induces physiologic changes opposite to "fight and flight," including reductions in blood pressure, heart rate, and serum cortisol levels. It is very easy to do, indeed the practice is inherently effortless. TM requires no particular lifestyle change or religious belief. However, because the technique is subtle, it requires in-person instruction from a qualified teacher. (Check www.tm.org for information and to find an instructor). In other words, TM is not something that you can learn on your own, casually from a friend, nor from a video or the internet. For patients with hypertension, TM has been shown effective in improving high blood pressure.[43,44] TM has likewise been found helpful in treating a range of other medical problems, including anxiety[45] and work-related stress.[46]

MBSR is an example of the open-monitoring type of meditation. Derived from Buddhist meditation traditions, the MBSR program was introduced at the University of Massachusetts Medical Center by Dr. Jon Kabat-Zinn in the late 1970s. Regarding MBSR, there is likewise a standardized and reproducible instruction format, a certification program for instructors, and widespread availability of instructors. Instruction can also be done online (www.umassmed.edu/cfm/mindfulness-based-programs). The practice of MBSR requires no specific religious beliefs. Mindfulness has been shown to be of help in managing a range of health-related disorders, including low back pain[47] and anxiety.[48]

Ideally you can add meditation practice to your routine twice daily, in the morning and afternoon. Wake up early, then meditate, then exercise. At midday, have a good lunch. Meditate late in the afternoon, and be certain to get to bed by 10 p.m. Next day, repeat, and so on. There you have it, the *picture of health!*

In addition to meditation, several movement or body-based techniques provide health benefits. These include yoga, tai chi, and qigong.

Yoga is a mind-body approach that aims to relieve stress and improve physical strength and flexibility. Regular yoga practice has been shown to be useful for pain management,[47,49] insomnia,[50] and other symptoms. One can generally find yoga instructors without difficulty in various studios or health clubs.

In traditional Chinese medicine, practitioners understand the concept "qi" as indicating the vital energy of life. Many of the therapeutics in Chinese medicine, such as acupuncture, aim to improve the flow of qi. There are also several mind-body approaches within the Chinese medicine tradition geared toward improving the flow of qi. These include qigong and tai chi. Tai Chi is a marital arts practice that has also been found to have health benefits. Tai Chi practice has been shown to be comparably effective to physical therapy for helping with arthritis[51] and to be effective in helping to improve cardiac function after a heart attack.[52] Tai Chi can also help to improve balance in patients with Parkinson disease.[53] Qigong techniques are of many types, generally combining movement and meditation. Scientists have shown qigong to be effective in managing high blood pressure,[54] and to be helpful with pain management.[55] You can find instructors in these techniques at various health clubs, community colleges and community centers, and through the offices of Chinese medicine practitioners.

In ayurveda, there is a concept called "behavioral rasayana." This refers to patterns of activity considered supportive of well-being and health. Examples of behavioral rasayanas include maintaining the company of wise and respected people, speaking in a way that is uplifting to others, and donating to charity. In addition, for those who adhere to a religious tradition, practicing one's own religion is held to be a behavioral rasayana of potential benefit to one's health. In the biomedical literature, for example, engaging in personal prayer[56] has been found to be associated with improvements in depression, anxiety, and coping. Along these lines, there exist traditions of meditation instruction and practice in all the great world religions, including Judaism,[57] Christianity,[58] and Islam.[59] Finally, scientists have documented that exposure to nature and wilderness environments helps to reduce stress and improve well-being.[60]

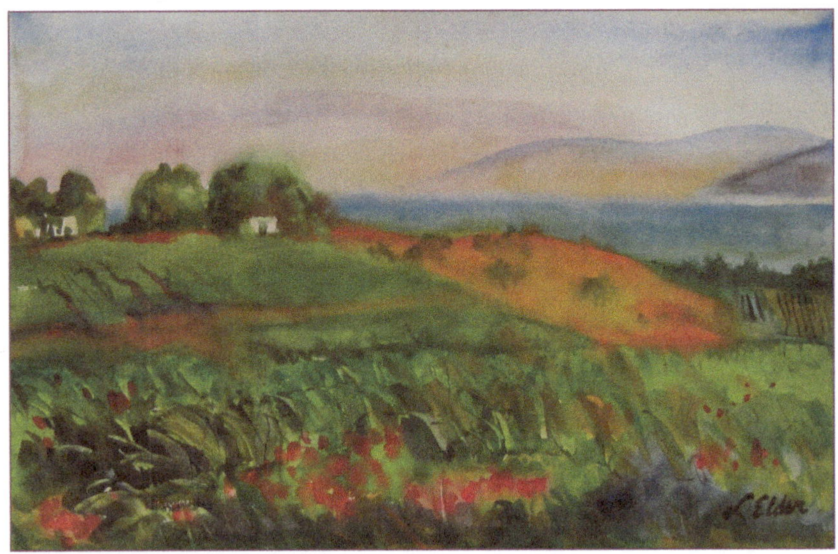

Lake Galilee
(watercolor)

Here is a view overlooking Lake Galilee, a precious resource that provides water for drinking and agriculture in a dry land. The area surrounding the lake encompasses sites holy to multiple religions.

The techniques and approaches reviewed in this chapter are experiential. Only so much can be usefully written about them because in the end they must be experienced. We provide our patients with an overview of what is available, and advice as to what might be helpful for the individual, on the basis of the patient's medical condition, personal preferences, and other circumstances. From there, we direct the patient toward available resources, and the ball is in his/her court! Regular practice of an authentic mind-body technique can significantly improve one's long-term health prospects. When we achieve quiet and peace of mind, we are setting the stage for the body to rebalance and heal. From the standpoint of ayurveda, regular meditation practice stabilizes and harmonizes the physiology at the most fundamental level, just as watering the root benefits the entire tree. As such, regular practice can be expected to promote balance of the doshas and overall health at all levels. In addition, meditation training provides a self-help tool that can be used indefinitely, empowering the patient to take control of his/her own health. Similarly, in Chinese medicine the aim of many practitioner-administered modalities, including acupuncture, is to balance the flow of qi, which is understood as the vital life force. Techniques like qigong likewise improve the flow of qi, but in this case we do not have a practitioner or supplement acting upon a passive patient. Instead, the patient gains a tool that places her in the cockpit in terms of improving and maintaining her health.

Patient Testimonials[61]

- *(Caregiver for spouse with history of stroke and severe motor vehicle accident)*
  "I was a caregiver; it was heavy duty ... I ended up in the emergency room three times and each time it was diagnosed as anxiety ... . There were panic attacks that were so much like heart attacks. I know that it was due to the stress of my caregiving role. I worried about him (my husband) constantly. I was always afraid of what would happen to him. TM helped me by just calming my thoughts ... it calmed me down and I could get through the day much easier. Since I have been doing TM I haven't had one anxiety attack ... this was the biggest benefit. I noticed less anxiety straight away."

- *(Caregiver for 92-year-old parent with dementia)*
  "I started TM two years ago ... the timing was perfect. I found it pretty easy and it made a lot of difference to me. I just felt calmer, I was much kinder to my mother, I didn't get as frustrated with her .... It's so hard when they can't do anything, they are like children and it is so frustrating because ... after a while you hit times where you just want to yell at them and it was so hard not to .... Then (through TM practice) I found that I didn't get like that as often; I found that I was more equalized, more balanced about it all. It was a very helpful tool. My mother has gotten worse but I am still able to do what needs to be done for her and be loving .... I gotta say that being able to deal with all that and not just falling apart really has to do with TM .... TM grows with you as you need more calm and more clarity of mind ... you need that more and more as they get worse and worse. TM is a tool that keeps on giving more and more."

CHAPTER EIGHT

DRUG, SUPPLEMENT, OR FOOD?

Which herbs work, which don't, and who's to say?

Scientists have derived a number of medications from plants. For example, most people are familiar with aspirin as a drug that has long been used for management of pain, inflammation, and fever. More recently, aspirin has also become an important medication as an antiplatelet agent to reduce risk of heart attack and stroke. As it turns out, aspirin has actually been around for a lot longer than most people realize.

The bark of the *willow tree* contains a chemical called salicin, which is very similar to aspirin in terms of both chemical structure and therapeutic effect.[62] Historical documents show that people used willow bark therapeutically for pain management in ancient Sumerian and Egyptian cultures as far back as 3500 years ago. Later, in ancient Greece, Hippocrates recommended willow bark to help with pain associated with childbirth. However, it wasn't until the 19th century that scientists eventually identified the active chemical ingredient in willow bark and gave it the name salicin. From there, over a period of decades, chemists modified the chemical structure of salicin first into a chemical called salicylic acid, and then, in 1897, into a new compound they named acetylsalicylic acid, which is the modern-day aspirin.

Most people think of aspirin as a drug, not as an herb, supplement, or food. However, in truth, scientists developed aspirin from a chemical originally identified as the active ingredient in a medicinal plant. Why not just use the plant?

For pain and inflammation, the use of aspirin as a drug offers many advantages over the use of willow bark. Pharmaceutical companies can patent drugs, but not plants, rendering their development, manufacture, and distribution more profitable. Modern consumers can therefore more easily find drugs than herbal supplements at the local pharmacy. Because scientists have identified and isolated an active ingredient, aspirin may be stronger, or more effective, and in a shorter period of time, relative to the plant. In addition, because aspirin has only one ingredient, companies can more reliably produce it in a pure and reproducible form, and physicians can more easily evaluate its efficacy in clinical trials.

Despite these advantages, many people prefer to use herbal supplements over drugs. What might be some of the reasons? Some people perceive herbal supplements as safer. In addition to the active ingredient or ingredients, the plant contains many other chemical constituents, which may serve to balance, or counteract, any potential side effects of the active ingredient. People thus perceive the herb as more gentle, with a more gradual onset of action. Nature produces the plant, not a laboratory. As such, the plant displays the same natural intelligence, or reflects the same blueprint, as our own physiology. In this respect many people believe the herb to be not only safer, but also more sustainable and effective in the long term. With drugs, because they are manmade or synthetic, our experience with them is relatively short. Indeed, we quite commonly learn about the unanticipated dangerous side effects of a drug as a few decades of experience accrue. Plants have been around more or less forever, and their effects, positive or negative, are, for the most part, well known.

Against this backdrop we can now examine how we can best use herbs and supplements to treat illness and to improve and maintain health. In ayurveda, naturopathy, Chinese medicine, and other holistic systems of medicine, the use of herbs, vitamins, and other supplements often play an important role in the treatment plan. But first, in an integrative medicine practice setting, there are several key issues to consider about the use of supplements.

First, *what proof, if any, exists to support the effectiveness of the supplement?* Scientists have shown many popular supplements, such as turmeric (for osteoarthritis), and feverfew (for migraine headaches), to be effective. At the same time, other popular supplements, such as Echinacea for the common cold, have not been found to be effective in clinical trials.[63] The use of some supplements in ayurveda, Chinese medicine, or Native American healing systems are supported by many thousands of years of experience. Many supplements have yet to be studied, or proved effective in clinical settings, yet there may be reason to think that the supplement could potentially be effective as one might infer from mechanistic studies done in animals.

Of major importance is the quality of the supplement: *Does the labelling on the bottle accurately reflect the contents?* There are 2 sides to this. First, does the product actually contain the specified ingredients as claimed? Second, is the product free of contaminants? One must keep in mind that in the United States, the Food and Drug Administration (FDA) does not regulate supplements with the same level of rigor as drugs, and labels may not accurately reflect the contents of the product. Therefore, it behooves the consumer to research and to identify a high-quality supplier. Many herbal products will have been inspected and certified by agencies or organizations beyond the FDA. For example, you can look for evidence of quality certifications such as USP (US Pharmacopeial Convention) (www.usp.org/verification-services), USDA organic, (www.usda.gov/topics/organic), ISO-9001 (www.iso.org/iso-9001-quality-management.html), and the National Formulary (NF) (USP-NF: www.usp.org/usp-nf). As another option for patients interested in a specific herbal product, you can contact the manufacturer directly and request a "certificate of analysis," detailing its contents.

Another important concern is the *safety of the product*. Even if the supplement contains precisely what is stated on the bottle, is this particular herb safe? Most herbal supplements are, but some are not. For example, regulators removed the supplement ephedra from the market in the United States because of potential safety concerns related to cardiovascular side effects. Likewise, they removed Kava from the market because of reports of liver toxicity. It is thus important to consider whether any particular supplement on the market is safe to take in the amount recommended. Reliable sources of information about safety and efficacy of herbal supplements include your physician or pharmacist, or on the Internet at the National Center for Complementary and Integrative Health (www.nccih.nih.gov), as well as Consumer Lab (www.consumerlab.com).

Another thing to consider is the possibility *of interactions between the herbal supplement and your medications and/or other supplements*. This may especially be of concern if you are taking a lot of medications, or if you have an upcoming surgical procedure. An herbal supplement could either potentiate, or block the effect or side effect of any drugs or supplements you are currently taking. An herbal supplement could also interact with a drug that may be administered as part of an upcoming procedure.

Next, *what is the cost of the supplement?* Sometimes companies charge a lot of money for supplements, so before spending a boatload of cash, you want to be certain that the potential benefits of the supplement justify the expenditure. There is a whole industry out there making a bundle of money selling vitamins and questionably useful supplements, frequently targeting elderly people. If a practitioner focuses on selling you large amounts of vitamins and supplements, promising you a rosy outcome if only you take his or her products, look for the door. When something sounds too good to be true, it usually is.

Finally, *have you discussed the situation with your physician and/or pharmacist*? It is always a good idea to review what supplements you are taking, or thinking about taking, with your physician, who can often advise you as to some of the pros and cons of any particular product, including efficacy, safety, and interactions. As a rule, we advise patients to discontinue all supplements 2 weeks before any planned surgical procedure. Your physician may also be able to discuss your use of supplements in the context of the bigger picture of your overall health.

Naturally, dealing with all these issues can sometimes be overwhelming for a patient. At Kaiser Permanente Northwest, a Natural Products Advisory Committee makes recommendations to the regional pharmacy as to which products to stock on our pharmacies' over-the-counter shelves.[64] After all, many patients are using supplements, and many physicians are recommending them. Sometimes, given all the pros and cons, after weighing safety, efficacy, quality, and cost, using a supplement often makes the most sense. We then stock these products on our over-the-counter pharmacy shelves as a convenience to our patients. In addition, our committee consists of a multidisciplinary team of physicians, pharmacists, dieticians, and other experts. Such a group can better research and identify a quality product for stocking, rather than leaving this difficult choice to the patient.

Following is a review of the supplements currently stocked on over-the-counter pharmacy shelves at Kaiser Permanente Northwest. These supplements may make sense for some patients to use, in consultation with a physician, as part of a treatment regimen for the specified condition.

MigreLief is a combination product providing 100 mg feverfew daily (50 mg taken twice daily) combined with 400 mg riboflavin plus 360 mg magnesium. Feverfew is a plant that has been found to be effective in preventing migraine headaches.[65] In addition, both magnesium (a mineral) and riboflavin (a B vitamin) have been found useful for preventing migraines. The MigreLief product simply combines all 3. Another approach a patient might reasonably take would be to purchase one or several of these ingredients individually, to be taken daily to help reduce the frequency of migraines. Although prescription drugs are available for migraine prevention, these may not be effective for, or may not be well tolerated by certain people.

St. John's Wort is a plant whose leaves and flowers are commonly used to treat mild to moderate depression. The usual dose is 300 mg 3 times a day of the extract standardized to 0.3% hypericin content. Studies have shown St. John's wort to be superior to placebo in patients with depression, and comparably effective to standard antidepressants, with fewer side effects.[66] Though appropriate for patients with moderate symptoms, people with severe depression, bipolar disorder, or schizophrenia should not rely on St. John's wort. Side effects may include photosensitivity, nausea, and dizziness. A significant drawback is the fact that St. John's wort has been associated with potentially serious interactions with a long list of medications. If you are using any other medications, it is best to consult with your physician or pharmacist before using St. John's wort.

Turmeric is a spice derived from the root of the turmeric plant. Turmeric has anti-inflammatory properties, and people use it for a wide range of indications. Scientists have shown turmeric to be helpful in treating pain caused by osteoarthritis.[67] As such, turmeric can be an effective and safe alternative to nonsteroidal anti-inflammatory medications (e.g., ibuprofen or naproxen) for this purpose. The adult dose is 500 mg 2 to 4 times daily. Common side effects include nausea and diarrhea. Turmeric may cause gallbladder contractions, and patients with gallstones or gallbladder disease should be cautious when using this supplement. Turmeric may interact with anticoagulant and antiplatelet drugs, and again must be used with caution, or in consultation with a physician, in this setting. Turmeric in high doses may stimulate menstrual blood flow and should be avoided in pregnancy.

Alpha lipoic acid is an antioxidant that is naturally synthesized by the body. Taking this supplement in a dose of 600 mg/day to 1200 mg/day can help reduce symptoms of painful neuropathy in people with diabetes.[68] Although the supplement is generally considered safe, potential side effects include hypoglycemia, reduced effectiveness of cancer chemotherapy, nausea, and skin rash.

Coenzyme Q10 is a compound naturally produced by the body that helps to facilitate a number of biochemical processes involved with energy metabolism. Some people believe that taking statin medications reduces the body's production of coenzyme Q10, and that this in turn causes the muscle aches and pains that people often report as a side effect of statin therapy. Taking a coenzyme Q10 supplement in a dose of 100 mg/day to 200 mg/day divided twice daily may be a good idea for people who need to take statin drugs to prevent or correct muscle pains. Some studies support this,[69] but the data have been inconsistent. Even so, the supplement is generally well tolerated, and may be of help for some patients who need to take statin drugs.

Melatonin is a hormone that is naturally produced by the pineal gland in the brain. Some evidence suggests that taken as a supplement, melatonin can help with both insomnia and jetlag.[70] People take a wide range of doses, typically from 0.5 mg to 5 mg. For jetlag, you should take the supplement at bedtime on arrival at your destination, continuing for 2 to 5 days. Side effects can include headache, transient depression, fatigue, cramps, and nausea. However, overall, people tolerate this supplement very well. Melatonin provides a good alternative to sleep medications that may have more frequent or serious side effects. You should avoid taking this supplement if you have high blood pressure, a seizure disorder, liver disease, or cerebral palsy.

Glucosamine is a substance normally produced by the body that is used to help build cartilage. Taken as a supplement, glucosamine sulfate can help with pain associated with osteoarthritis. Research findings are somewhat contradictory,[71] but on balance this can be a relatively safe alternative to nonsteroidal anti-inflammatory drugs for some patients with chronic pain caused by osteoarthritis. The usual dose is 500 mg 3 times a day. Patients with shellfish allergy must avoid this supplement. Although glucosamine sulfate is usually well tolerated, side effects can include gastrointestinal distress and headache.

Consumption of **fish oils** has been shown to be associated with reduced risk of cardiovascular disease,[72] and in higher doses, is effective for reducing serum triglycerides. The active fatty acids in fish oils are eicosapentaenoic acid (EPA) and docosahexaenoic acid (DHA). Recommended doses for cardiovascular disease prevention are 1400 mg EPA + DHA per day. For lowering serum triglycerides, the recommended dosing is 2000-3000 mg EPA + DHA per day. Fish oil supplementation is safe and is a good idea for people at risk for developing heart disease. For those on a vegetarian diet, or who otherwise wish to avoid consuming fish oils, flaxseed oil provides an alternative. However, as a supplement for reducing cardiovascular risk, the fatty acids in flax seed oil are not as effective as those found in fish oils.

Probiotics are living microorganisms, like bacteria or yeast, that can have a beneficial effect on health. Probiotics are found in many foods, including yogurt products, and can also be taken as a supplement. There are different types of probiotic supplements that are available on the market, the most common of which include *Lactobacillus* or

Bifidobacterium species. The mechanism by which probiotics improve health is not clear but could involve promotion of a protective barrier to prevent harmful organisms or materials from crossing from the intestinal tract into the bloodstream. Healthful bacteria in the colon are also thought to play a beneficial role in promoting immune function. Taking probiotics may be effective in reducing the duration of diarrheal illnesses,[73] in preventing diarrhea associated with antibiotics,[74] in improving symptoms of irritable bowel,[75] and for other conditions. Dosing will vary, depending on the preparation.

Zinc lozenges can be helpful in the treatment of symptoms of common cold.[76] The suggested dose is 12 mg every 2 hours at onset of cold symptoms. However, sometimes patients have difficulty tolerating zinc, because of side effects such as bad taste and nausea.

Cranberry concentrate has been found to be effective in reducing the occurrence of urinary tract infections.[77] The recommended dose of cranberry concentrate capsules is 500 mg 1 to 2 times a day. Another option is to use a cranberry juice cocktail (such us Ocean Spray, which provides 26% cranberry juice) 300 mL (10 ounces) daily. Cranberry is safe and well tolerated. The mechanism of action involves interference with bacterial attachment to urinary tract epithelial cells.

Peppermint has been found to be effective in managing symptoms of irritable bowel syndrome.[78] Scientists have found that taking enteric-coated peppermint oil reduces abdominal pain, distention, and other symptoms. Side effects can include abdominal pain or nausea. The usual dose is 1 to 2 capsules 3 times daily of enteric-coated peppermint oil (with each capsule providing approximately 180 mg to 225 mg peppermint oil).

A number of other herbal products are popular, but some of these we have elected not to stock at Kaiser Permanente Northwest pharmacies owing to concerns about safety or evidence. Examples include Echinacea (for the common cold), and black cohosh (for menopausal symptoms). Other supplements have been stocked in the past, but later discontinued as new information questioning their efficacy became available. Examples include saw palmetto (for prostatic symptoms) as well as gingko biloba (for cognitive insufficiency).

The following 3 supplements are commonly used in ayurveda, and we often recommend them in our practice. These may be useful as single-ingredient supplements for some patients.

Boswellia, also known as Indian frankincense, is an herbal supplement commonly used to treat musculoskeletal pain and inflammation. Studies have shown improvements in pain and inflammation for patients with arthritis.[79] Boswellia is usually well tolerated. Dosing will vary depending on the preparation.

Brahmi, also known as Bacopa, is an herbal supplement regarded in ayurveda as beneficial for optimizing mental functioning and managing mental stress. Patients take 2 g to 4 g of the whole plant daily in divided doses. Some scientific evidence supports the use of Brahmi for the traditional indications. In one study,[80] healthy adults taking a Brahmi supplement, compared with those taking placebo, showed improvements in memory acquisition and retention. Reported gastrointestinal side effects included increased stool frequency, abdominal cramps, and nausea

Ashwagandha is an adaptogen that helps the body to resist stress. According to ayurveda, it increases stamina and energy and improves overall well-being. Ashwaganda is an excellent herb for balancing vata dosha. Suggested dose of the root is 1 g to 2 g per day. In one study, investigators recruited 64 people with chronic stress[81] and randomly assigned participants to receive either the herbal supplement or a placebo. Those who took the actual supplement showed improvements in both stress assessment scales and serum cortisol levels. Ashwagandha is very well tolerated in the usual doses.

In summary, on the basis of clinical trial evidence, a number of herbs and supplements appear to be safe and effective in certain clinical circumstances. This information is of high importance, but herbal medicine is a vast topic, and we have only begun to scratch the surface.

Across medical systems, practitioners, and patients, people think about the use of herbal supplements from a range of perspectives. Should we think of supplements as drugs, or as foods, or as something in between? On the one side, many view supplements through the same lens through which we view pharmaceuticals. As already discussed, we derived many drugs used today from plants, including aspirin, morphine, digoxin, and others. By this line of thinking, we use herbs to treat specific medical conditions just as we do drugs. We can evaluate the efficacy of these herbs using the same research strategies that are applied to evaluating pharmaceuticals, and we can even isolate the active ingredient of the plant, manufacture it in a laboratory, and sell it as a drug.

The understanding of the total nature of the subject does not arise from a fragmentary knowledge of it.
— Charaka Samhita, Vimanasthana 4.5

Further along the continuum would be a whole plant, or an intact part of the plant (such as the root or leaves). In such instances, the practitioner prepares or prescribes an herb or herbal part as a whole entity. S/he makes no effort to isolate an active chemical ingredient. Instead, the active ingredient or ingredients in the plant are present, along with many other chemical constituents. We may expect the supplement to have a clinical effect less immediate or dramatic compared with a drug, but potentially with far less risk in terms of toxicity or side effects, as other components of the plant may help balance the properties of the active ingredients. Although we can still prescribe, or study, a particular plant for a particular medical problem in this way, the situation is starting to get a little murky. We don't know with certainty what the active ingredient or ingredients are, nor can we be confident that the concentration of these ingredients remains consistent from one crop of the plant to the next. People use herbs in this way, but from a conventional scientific perspective, it is harder to draw conclusions.

Somewhere in the middle are the standardized herbal extracts, like St. John's wort or Gingko biloba. Scientists identify a presumptive active ingredient and produce an herbal extract containing a standardized amount of this compound. In the case of St. John's wort, this would be the extract standardized to 0.3% hypericin content. The manufacturer has included a specified amount of this active ingredient in the preparation; however, other ingredients from the plant, in unspecified amounts, remain. Here, we expect the trade-off in terms of potency and side effects to be intermediate between that of a drug on the one hand, and the intact plant on the other.

To further complicate the story, in ayurveda and other complementary medicine systems, we commonly prescribe herbal mixtures. One well-known example is *triphala,* a mixture of three herbs. Triphala acts as a mild laxative and as a *rasayana,* or tonic, to promote health and treat a range of health disorders. Alternatively, practitioners may formulate an herbal mixture to help treat a particular condition. Of course, an herbalist does not just randomly toss a bunch of ingredients together. Rather, ayurveda describes a sophisticated system of herbal energetics that guides the preparation of each formula. Just as we analyze foods in terms of their tastes and qualities, in ayurveda we assess herbs in terms of taste, potency (heating or cooling), aftertaste, and other special properties. In addition, an herbalist may include specific ingredients in an herbal mixture for any number of reasons. An herb may function as an active or therapeutic ingredient, or may potentiate the effect of other active ingredients in the formula. Alternatively, an herbal ingredient may serve to counteract potential side effects of the active ingredients in the formula, or may function to facilitate the delivery of the active ingredients to the physiology. Sometimes, in ayurveda, naturopathy, or Chinese medicine, the practitioner will adjust the ingredients of the herbal formula after a period of treatment, in response to the progress of the patient.

If a scientist wants to do a clinical trial evaluating the efficacy of an herbal preparation, how can s/he possibly draw any conclusions if the supplement has multiple ingredients whose relative proportions are in a state of flux? We have looked at research on single herbs, or herbal extracts, but from the complementary and integrative medicine perspective, using herbs in this way isn't always appropriate. In the real world, we often prescribes mixtures of herbs, basing their formulation on a non-Western paradigm, and adjusting their concentrations on the basis of the patient's clinical response to therapy.

On top of that, from a complementary and integrative medicine standpoint, we might not prescribe an herbal supplement in isolation, either as a single or multi-ingredient preparation, but rather within the context of a multimodality protocol. We recommend the herbs along with a broader program of dietary adjustments, lifestyle changes, mind-body instruction, exercise, and other types of modalities, all intended to work together in synergy. Indeed, from the standpoint of ayurvedic theory, we might not even *expect* an herbal to be useful in and of itself if the patient is not following a reasonable diet and routine.

Finally, many of the herbs used in ayurveda, such as turmeric and ginger, commonly serve as spices that we frequently cook with. We have already emphasized the importance of including these spices in the diet.

Bitter gourd is a plant used in ayurveda to help lower blood sugars. You can slice it up and cook it as a food with your stir-fry, or drink the juice, or use it as a supplement, or all three.

Considering all this flips our thinking upside down. When we do clinical trials of herbal preparations, we generally assume a paradigm that conceptualizes the supplement as though it were a drug. To properly analyze supplements from the standpoint of the complementary medicine system, we must think more in terms of herbal energetics, taking into account the synergy of multiple modalities, and the effectiveness of the overall clinical paradigm (see Chapter Ten). This is a much more difficult scenario to consider in the context of biomedical research. Some studies in the literature have, in fact, evaluated the effectiveness of multimodality complementary medicine protocols that include but are not limited to herbs,[82] but much more research is needed in this area.

Patients and physicians both need to be savvy, and more patient-physician dialogue is always better than less. Patients should remember that while supplements can play an important part in a treatment or health maintenance program, they do not substitute for proper diet, exercise, and routine. In addition, we generally advise patients to limit the number of herbal supplements to no more than 3 or 4. Taking more than that only confuses things. Patients should use supplements only under the guidance of a physician and/or a complementary medicine practitioner. People should avoid self-medicating. Mixtures of herbs prescribed by a licensed practitioner generally cause fewer problems and less concern than those off the shelf in the context of self-medicating. Patients already taking lots of medications need to exercise caution when it comes to adding supplements, and those taking certain medications, for example blood thinners such as warfarin, must avoid supplements altogether. Transplant patients taking immunosuppressive medications should likewise avoid supplements.

Physicians and pharmacists should ask their patients about the supplements they are taking while maintaining a constructive and supportive tone to the dialogue. In other words, any discussion of herbal supplements should not lead the patient to a dead end. Some health care professionals make the mistake of retreating to a maximally conservative position, advising patients to avoid all supplements, altogether, all the time. In some circumstances, this may be the right advice, but at other times such comments may be counterproductive. Rejecting the patient's interest in supplements can worsen the situation by detracting from confidence in the physician/patient relationship, and by discouraging the patient from using interventions of potential therapeutic benefit. In contrast, thoughtfully encouraging self-care improves patient morale and empowers the patient to participate in his/her own care.

Finally, we have talked at length about herbal supplements, but what about vitamins? Generally speaking, a good-balanced diet provides the nutrients we need, and taking lots of vitamin supplements should be unnecessary. Vitamin D comes from sun exposure rather than the diet, meaning that a Vitamin D supplement is a good idea for those in locations where sun exposure is limited. Patients following a vegan diet must take a Vitamin B_{12} supplement by mouth in doses of 1 mg a day (vitamin B_{12} injections are usually unnecessary). Postmenopausal women should take not only Vitamin D, but also a calcium supplement, in the amount of 1000 mg to 1500 mg daily.

Beyond that, if you want to take a single multivitamin tablet a day there is no harm done, but there is little reason to think that doing so is of much benefit.[83]

CHAPTER NINE

IS ACUPUNCTURE JUST PLACEBO?

Do acupuncture, chiropractic manipulation, and massage work for pain management? Explore what's really behind the science.

Acupuncture is a popular intervention, especially for chronic pain. A lot of people will tell you that it works. Is it really true, or is acupuncture just placebo?

Before answering this question, let's first discuss what we mean by "placebo." The word comes from the Latin verb "*placere*," meaning "to please." According to the Merriam-Webster dictionary,[84] a placebo is defined as "a usually pharmacologically inert preparation prescribed more for the mental relief of the patient than for its actual effect on a disorder." However, this definition implies that mental health problems are not actual disorders, which of course is not the case. In addition, because mind and body are connected, the mental relief of the patient could possibly affect the outcome of a physical illness. Unfortunately, the dictionary definition introduces too many problems to be of use, so we will need to explore for ourselves exactly what is meant by the term "placebo."

Next, what do we mean by "acupuncture"? Again, per Merriam-Webster,[84] acupuncture can be defined as "an originally Chinese practice of inserting fine needles through the skin at specific points, especially to cure disease or relieve pain." This definition likewise presents problems. First, some styles of acupuncture practice prescribe application of pressure at acupoints without actual needle insertion. Second, there is a practice in conventional medicine called dry needling, in which the physician inserts needles into connective tissues to relieve pain. Most physicians who perform dry needling wouldn't consider it to be acupuncture.

Clearly, this dictionary definition, too, is lacking, and we find ourselves heading for murky waters.

In addressing the question, "Is acupuncture just placebo?", we will adopt a unique approach. Specifically, we will review in detail 3 important studies that scientists have published in this area. This review in turn will empower us to answer our question in a way that does adequate justice to the complexity and nuance of the issue.

If you have less interest in the scientific data, you can just skim this chapter and get the main points by reviewing the "highlights" section. If you want to use acupuncture but your physician is skeptical, *make sure your physician reads the entire chapter!*

What's In A Placebo?

The first study[85] was a project done by researchers at Harvard involving patients with irritable bowel syndrome. The investigators proposed an interesting idea. They suggested that the placebo effect, as we generally talk about it, really has 3 separate components. In other words, when people reference the placebo effect, they may be thinking about 1 or more of 3 different phenomena that often get jumbled up or confused. The first component of the placebo effect is the effect of being observed. We call this the Hawthorne effect. People you pay attention to behave differently simply because they know you are paying attention to them. In research, patients enrolled in a study behave differently from those who are not enrolled in the study. In clinical practice, the patients that physicians pay attention to behave differently from those patients that physicians ignore. In sum, paying attention to a patient can influence that person's behavior and clinical outcomes. This is the first component of the placebo effect.

The second component of the placebo effect is the patient's response to the performance of some therapeutic ritual. For example, the "ritual" of inserting acupuncture needles, or of writing a prescription, or of performing a medical procedure, can potentially impress and encourage a patient, and thus influence the outcome.

The third component of the placebo effect is the impact of the physician-patient relationship. A good relationship between patient and physician can improve clinical outcomes. Along these lines, when the physician projects positive expectations for a good outcome, this can become a self-fulfilling prophecy.

Kaptchuk et al[85] proposed that the placebo effect can be divided into the 3 aforementioned components, and that each component can then be added one to another incrementally, to achieve better and better responses. In other words, they hypothesized that they could provide component 1 of the placebo effect and achieve improvement in their patients, then add to that the second component to get an even better effect, then finally add to that the third component to get an even better outcome still.

To test this they recruited 262 people suffering from symptoms of irritable bowel syndrome. Patients who signed up for the study completed questionnaires at enrollment, then at week 3 and at week 6. These questionnaires collected information about severity and relief of symptoms and overall quality of life. Kaptchuk et al[85] assigned each study participant at random to 1 of 3 groups. The people in the first group served as a "wait list control." This means that they enrolled in the study, but aside from completing the questionnaires every few weeks, nothing more was done with them. There was no intervention. Thus this group received the first component of the placebo effect only. They were under observation, but that's it.

For it is good remedy sometimes to apply nothing at all.
— Hippocrates

The second group was called the "limited placebo" group. This group received a set of placebo, or sham, acupuncture treatments, but it was predetermined in advance that they would not enjoy a meaningful relationship with the acupuncturist. These sham acupuncture treatments took place twice a week during the course of the study. Usually, a practitioner inserts acupuncture needles into specific acupoints on the skin, but for the sham treatments the acupuncturist used points on the skin that are not known acupoints. In addition, the acupuncturist didn't actually insert the needles. Instead, s/he used a sham acupuncture device that created the illusion of penetrating the skin by retracting into a hollow handle. Prior experience had shown this device to be effective at fooling patients into believing that they were receiving real acupuncture.

Beyond the sham acupuncture, the participants assigned to this group did not get much else from the acupuncturist. The practitioner spent little time with each patient, and explained that s/he had been instructed not to talk to the patient. The practitioner would place the sham "needles," and then leave the patient alone for about 20 minutes with the sham devices in place. Then the practitioner returned to remove the sham "needles." Subsequent visits proceeded in similar fashion.

Participants in this limited placebo group received 2 of the 3 components of the placebo effect. They were enrolled and being measured in the study, and they were receiving a therapeutic ritual (sham acupuncture), but they still lacked a meaningful relationship with the practitioner.

The third intervention group in this study was called the "augmented placebo" group. This group was enrolled in the study, and received the sham acupuncture ritual. In addition, these participants also experienced a high-quality interaction with the acupuncture practitioner. The initial visit with the acupuncturist was a full 45 minutes in length, and was structured with respect to both content and style. Content of the discussion included questions about symptoms, the impact and meaning of the condition on the patient, and the like. The practitioner also included behaviors such as a friendly manner, active listening, empathy, communication of positive expectations for treatment result, and thoughtful silence while taking the pulse. Only after completing this checklist of content and behaviors did the practitioner then place the sham acupuncture devices.

Participants in this third group received all 3 components of the placebo effect. They were enrolled in the study, added to that they received the therapeutic ritual, and added on top of all that they also enjoyed a quality relationship with the practitioner.

In the end, what happened? How did the groups do in comparison with one another? The data showed that for each of the 4 outcome measures, those in the wait list group improved, those in the limited group improved more and those in the augmented group improved most of all. In summary, placebo worked! The more components of the placebo that were applied, the better the effect! In addition, the data showed that participants got the most "bang for the buck" with the addition of the augmented practitioner relationship.

What are the take-home lessons? First, when people talk about placebo effects they are often mixing up several different phenomena. When someone claims that "acupuncture is just placebo," what does s/he mean by "placebo"? Is s/he talking about the effect of observing the patient, or the effect of a therapeutic ritual, or the impact of the practitioner-patient relationship, or some combination of the above? Second, placebo works. The patients in all the groups got better over time. If our goal is to make patients feel better, then if placebo is going to do the trick, is that so bad? Finally, the data suggest that the relationship between physician and patient, and the attitudes we all bring to the clinical encounter, influence outcomes. When the physician and/or patient approach a therapy with a positive attitude, this favorably impacts the outcome, and vice versa.

STUDIES SHOW THAT PLACEBOS WORK!
A physician can use placebo effects to better help the patient.

How Do Different Types Of Acupuncture Compare?

Now that we have a better sense as to what we mean by "placebo" effects, let's look at another study,[86] this time evaluating various forms of acupuncture for low back pain. This project took place at Group Health Cooperative in the Puget Sound area (now Kaiser Permanente Washington) and at Kaiser Permanente in Northern California. A total of 641 patients with chronic low back pain enrolled in the study. The research team assigned each of the patients at random to 1 of 4 treatment groups: usual care, individualized acupuncture, standardized acupuncture, and simulated acupuncture. All patients completed questionnaires at study enrollment, then 8 weeks later, 26 weeks later, and 52 weeks later. These questionnaires gathered information about disability, symptom bothersomeness, and other outcomes.

Those assigned to the usual care group received usual care, and that was it. They went about their business in the health care system as usual. All patients assigned to one of the acupuncture groups saw a diagnosing acupuncturist, who evaluated the patient and provided a Chinese medicine diagnosis. The diagnosing acupuncturist also prescribed an individualized acupuncture treatment protocol to each patient on the basis of this Chinese medicine diagnosis. Each of the patients in the 3 acupuncture groups then went to see the treating acupuncturist twice weekly for 3 weeks, and then weekly for 4 weeks, for a total of 10 treatments over about 7 weeks. All patients receiving acupuncture wore eye masks and lay prone with their face in a cradle during treatments, so they couldn't see what the acupuncturist was actually doing.

The acupuncturist treated those participants assigned to the individualized acupuncture group using the individualized acupuncture protocol constructed specifically for that patient on the basis of the Chinese medicine diagnosis. In contrast, the acupuncturist treated those in the standardized acupuncture group with a one-size-fits-all standardized acupuncture protocol. This was a general pre-set group of acupoints considered by acupuncture experts to be effective for back pain.

Why did the investigators include separate groups for individualized and standardized acupuncture? In traditional Chinese medicine, practitioners generally prescribe individualized treatment regimens on the basis of the Chinese medicine diagnosis. Low back pain is a conventional medicine diagnosis. Patients with low back pain may fall into a variety of diagnostic categories from a Chinese medicine standpoint, and so perhaps they shouldn't all be treated in the same way. If you do treat all comers alike, on the basis of the conventional medicine diagnosis, then some patients may receive suboptimal treatment, and the study could miss, or underestimate, the treatment effect. On the other hand, from the standpoint of logistics it is much easier to provide just one treatment protocol for everyone with low back pain. One of the things the investigators wanted to do in this study was to determine whether individualizing the acupuncture treatment protocol on the basis of Chinese medicine diagnostics actually made any difference in improving the outcomes.

The third acupuncture group was the sham or placebo acupuncture group. When treating these patients, the practitioner used the same set of acupoints that were used in the standardized acupuncture treatment protocol. However, the acupuncturist did not actually insert the needles. Instead, he used a toothpick in a needle guide tube. The acupuncturist gently tapped and twisted this toothpick over the skin. This third group provided the sham, or placebo, control group to see if there would be any effect of "real" acupuncture above and beyond this "placebo" acupuncture intervention.

How did the various groups do? At 8 weeks, at the completion of acupuncture treatments, all groups had improved their disability scores. In addition, all 3 of the acupuncture groups improved significantly more than the usual care group, but the investigators found no significant difference between the 3 acupuncture groups. Interestingly, although treatment stopped at week 8, the functional improvements in the acupuncture groups over usual care persisted and remained significant a year out! The pattern of results for symptom bothersomeness was similar. The investigators also found a reduction in the use of pain medications for those receiving acupuncture compared with usual care.

So, what do we conclude from this study? Is acupuncture just placebo? Advocates will point to the fact that all 3 acupuncture groups did better than the usual care groups, and will use the data to argue that acupuncture works. Skeptics will note that "real" acupuncture was no better than the "sham" acupuncture, and use the data to argue that acupuncture is "just placebo." Others may not care whether the improved outcomes in this study were caused by placebo effects or not. The important thing is that acupuncture worked, by whatever mechanism, and the effect was durable.

> When comparing acupuncture to other types of interventions, many studies have shown that acupuncture works for pain management.

Finally, perhaps the sham acupuncture intervention in this study wasn't really a placebo. Maybe even the sham acupuncture had at least some therapeutic effect. We mentioned that in some systems of acupuncture practitioners only apply pressure, but don't actually penetrate the skin with the needle. Perhaps just applying pressure to the acupoint was enough to provide clinical benefit. Bear in mind that from a conventional medicine perspective we don't understand how acupuncture works. Because we don't know what the active ingredient is, we can't know with any certainty whether the "placebo" intervention included this active ingredient or not.

What If You Combine The Data?

Thus far, we have looked at one study that showed that placebos work, but that the placebo effect has multiple components to it. We then looked at another study showing that acupuncture was better than usual care for low back pain, although the investigators found no differences between sham, individualized, or standardized acupuncture. Let's review one last study to help clear things up. This last study was a "meta-analysis."[87] A meta-analysis is a study of studies. In a meta-analysis the investigators take a group of studies that have already been done on a particular topic and combine them to look at all the data in aggregate. By combining all the studies on a given topic, they gain a much larger number of patients to analyze. This allows scientists to see patterns in the overall data that may not be evident in the individual studies. In addition, with such a large dataset, people may be able to pick up on findings that were too small to detect in the smaller individual projects.

For this analysis, Vickers et al[87] combined all the data from 29 studies of acupuncture for chronic pain into 1 big data set that encompassed 17,922 patients. They analyzed data from high-quality studies of acupuncture for patients with 4 chronic pain conditions, including back and neck pain, osteoarthritis, chronic headache, and shoulder pain. For each condition they conducted 2 sets of comparisons. They compared patients who received acupuncture with patients who received sham acupuncture, and they also compared patients who received acupuncture with those who did not receive acupuncture. The results of the combined analyses were very interesting. Vickers et al[87] found that in the combined data sets, acupuncture was superior to no acupuncture for all of the conditions evaluated. In addition, in the combined datasets, they found that for all the conditions tested, acupuncture was also better than sham acupuncture! This was an important finding. The study provided the first robust data in the biomedical literature showing that "real" acupuncture was better than "sham" acupuncture. The authors were able to demonstrate this by combining the data from multiple smaller studies together.

Let's look at the comparative effect sizes reported in the paper. First, what is an effect size? This is a way of quantifying the difference between 2 groups. There are different ways of defining what an effect size is, but in general you take the difference in outcome between the two groups, and divide by the "standard deviation" (i.e., the overall spread) in the set of values. In other words, the greater the difference between the 2 groups in terms of outcome, the greater the effect size. The greater the variability, or spread, in the data, however, the lower the effect size. Generally speaking, people consider an effect size of 2 to be a "small" effect size, whereas 0.5 represents a "medium" effect size and 0.8 a "large" effect size.

Vickers et al[87] reported that the effect sizes for acupuncture vs no acupuncture were generally larger than those for acupuncture vs sham. For example, for osteoarthritis, the effect size is 0.26 for acupuncture vs sham, as opposed to 0.57 for acupuncture vs no acupuncture. This suggests that some of the effects of acupuncture are caused by "placebo" effects, but not all. The effect size for acupuncture vs sham are small but still significant, showing that once the "placebo" effects are accounted for, we still see a significant effect of acupuncture treatment.

Combining the data from the best studies, scientists showed that real acupuncture works better than placebo acupuncture.

In sum, is acupuncture just placebo? The scientific data suggest that the answer is no. Placebo accounts for part, but not all, of the effect of acupuncture. In addition, the effects of acupuncture for back pain are lasting. In the Cherkin study,[86] an 8-week course of acupuncture led to effects persisting almost a year later.

As data such as these are published, acupuncture has achieved increasing acceptance as a complementary medicine approach for helping to care for patients, and conventional medicine practitioners commonly refer patients to acupuncturists to help with chronic pain. Data also show acupuncture to be effective not only for chronic pain, but also for managing nausea and vomiting associated with cancer chemotherapy or pregnancy, as well as for urinary incontinence. Physicians at Kaiser Permanente Northwest can refer patients to acupuncturists in the community for any of these indications. Acupuncture may be effective for other conditions as well, but the data are less certain.

Kaiser Permanente Northwest physicians refer patients to acupuncturists not only for help with chronic pain, but also for managing nausea and vomiting associated with cancer chemotherapy or pregnancy, as well as for urinary incontinence.

What About Chiropractic Care And Massage?

Manual therapies, such as *chiropractic care,* are also effective, and commonly used, for the management of musculoskeletal pain.[88] The strongest evidence is for back and neck pain, and physicians at Kaiser Permanente Northwest frequently refer patients with back and neck pain to chiropractors to help manage their care. Data support the use of m*assage therapy* for low back pain as well.[89]

Kaiser Permanente Northwest physicians commonly refer patients to chiropractors to help with back and neck pain.

WHAT DO PATIENTS AND PHYSICIANS HAVE TO SAY ABOUT ACUPUNCTURE?[90]

Patients report the following:

[Acupuncture] helps me to be me. Doing drugs, I'm not the same person. … Since seeing an acupuncturist [for the last 5 months] I'm completely off every medication I've ever been on.

I actually had an appointment [with the pain clinic] and was waiting for months. But in the meantime, I had started acupuncture. And so by the time I was seen, I actually didn't need any additional pain meds or anything.

Physicians report the following:

I've seen so many of my patients who really get relief from nothing else, but get decent relief from [acupuncture]. … You see a patient [after they've had acupuncture] and they look better. They look relaxed. You don't see the little furrow between the brows … they can say to you, oh well, yeah, I have better range of motion. But it's more than just that. It's just a sense of, 'I feel better.'

I would be more likely to support and refer [to acupuncture], than to use even some of our most long-standing meds that we've used every day in a patient for years. […] it's that weighing of, what are my options that are relatively safe for this patient?

CHAPTER TEN

MODALITY OR SYSTEM?

Naturopathy, homeopathy, functional medicine, and more. Why is it so difficult for your primary care physician and naturopath to work together, and what can be done about it?

We have reviewed a number of complementary medicine modalities that improve the care of our patients. These include not only diet and exercise, but also daily routine, mind-body techniques, herbal and nutritional supplements, acupuncture, chiropractic manipulation, and more. Each of these modalities can enhance well-being and health, but there is more here than meets the eye.

If you visit a Chinese medicine practitioner, s/he may treat you with acupuncture. However, s/he may also include a variety of other modalities as part of your treatment regimen. These might include herbs, diet, moxibustion, and/or qigong, all in combination with acupuncture. In the same way, when providing an integrative ayurvedic consultation, we seldom prescribe only herbs. Our recommendations typically span a range of modalities, including not only herbs but also diet, daily routine, exercise, meditation, and more.

In this chapter we will review several additional systems of complementary and integrative medicine, including naturopathy. Each of these systems may prescribe a variety of modalities, alone or in combination, but can differ in terms of rationale, style, and emphasis. If you like, you can just skim this chapter and get the main points by reviewing the "highlights" section. If you are seeing a naturopathic physician, *ask both your primary care physician and your naturopath to read the entire chapter!*

When we think about acupuncture as an individual modality, and study it that way in a clinical trial, it is a little artificial. Rather than asking if acupuncture works, shouldn't we be asking if Chinese medicine works? When the practitioner treats the patient with all the relevant modalities from the Chinese medicine system in combination, what is the cumulative treatment effect? In the end, this is the most clinically relevant point. What results accrue not from applying an artificially isolated individual modality, but rather from implementing the *whole system* of care in managing the patient? This is a much tougher question to evaluate, and little such data are available. Research in Chinese medicine has focused mostly on acupuncture, and mostly for chronic pain. Yet Chinese medicine has a long history of use, with potential for applications in integrative medicine settings beyond just acupuncture for chronic pain. Perhaps when practiced as a whole, authentic, multimodality system, the applications of Chinese medicine could prove much broader.

When discussing complementary and integrative medicine, we must thus distinguish between modalities, like acupuncture or herbs, and whole systems of care characterized by a unique approach to the patient and encompassing a variety of such modalities. We have talked at length about one system of care, ayurveda, and how we apply the paradigm in guiding our use of a number of modalities, including diet, daily routine, exercise, mind-body techniques, and herbs. We have mentioned another system of care, traditional Chinese medicine, and reviewed in detail one of its most popular modalities, acupuncture. What about other medical systems?

One system that is widely practiced and used in North America is *naturopathy*. What exactly is naturopathy?

According to the House of Delegates position paper from the American Association of Naturopathic Physicians,[91] "Naturopathic medicine is a distinct method of primary health care—an art, science, philosophy, and practice of diagnosis, treatment, and prevention of illness." In stark contrast to a narrowly interpreted biomedical model where pharmaceuticals are administered to battle disease, "Naturopathic physicians seek to restore and maintain optimum health in their patients by emphasizing nature's inherent self-healing process … . This is accomplished through education and the rational use of natural therapeutics."[91] The naturopathic physician thus aims to use holistic approaches to enhance and restore the body's own innate healing systems. Naturopaths undergo a 4-year graduate-level course of study but are generally not residency trained. The American Association of Naturopathic Medical Colleges includes 8 institutions in North America, 3 of which are in the Pacific Northwest. Currently, in the US, licensing laws for naturopathic physicians exist in 19 states and the District of Columbia.[92]

Naturopathy is most accurately viewed as a whole system of medical practice,[93] representing not a distinct modality, but rather a paradigm guiding the selection and prescription of relatively complex, individualized, multimodality treatment regimens. However, in contrast to traditional Chinese medicine, which the conventional medicine community reduces to acupuncture, and chiropractic care, which the conventional medicine community reduces to spinal manipulation, naturopathy has defied reduction to a single modality. This has rendered naturopathy both difficult to study in clinical trial settings and more challenging to integrate into conventional medical treatment algorithms.

Naturopathy represents a unique approach to the patient, and cannot be reduced to a single modality. This makes it more difficult to do studies of naturopathy, and to integrate naturopathy with conventional care.

Nevertheless, naturopathy is popular among patients, and is widely used, for a number of reasons. For one, patients want a more holistic style of care, and naturopathic physicians can step in to fill that void. Naturopathic physicians are licensed in many parts of North America and patients can readily access them. Washington state law actually requires health insurers to cover naturopathy when medically indicated. Specifically, there is a statute in Washington that requires insurance companies to provide coverage for any category of licensed health care practitioner. In practice, because Washington licenses naturopaths, Kaiser Permanente and other health insurers operating in the state must, by law, provide coverage for naturopathic care when medically appropriate. In response, Kaiser Permanente Northwest has developed medical necessity criteria to define when naturopathic care may be medically indicated. The usual approach to the development of such criteria would be a systematic evaluation of efficacy data from randomized controlled trials (RCT). Such evidence reviews have been conducted in the development of medical necessity criteria for both acupuncture and chiropractic manipulation and are regularly updated. However, because naturopathy defines not a single modality but rather a paradigm, there is little such RCT data in the literature, and thus the evidence review toward defining medical necessity criteria for naturopathy required a modified, evidence-informed approach. To accomplish this, we queried leading naturopathic physicians in our community to identify those conditions they considered most appropriate for naturopathic referral. We then searched the literature across each of these conditions for evidence of efficacy for individual modalities commonly prescribed in naturopathy, such as diet, herbals, counseling, exercise, and stress reduction. The resulting "evidence grid" provided a picture of where naturopathic care could potentially be expected to be effective.

Physicians at Kaiser Permanente Northwest can refer patients for naturopathic care for any of several conditions, including osteoarthritis, menopausal symptoms, irritable bowel syndrome, headache, chronic fatigue, and eczema.

Currently, Kaiser Permanente Northwest will refer patients for naturopathic care who have failed usual care for any of several conditions, including osteoarthritis, menopausal symptoms, irritable bowel syndrome, headache, chronic fatigue, and eczema.

In addition, considerable anecdotal evidence supports the notion that naturopathic care often benefits these patients. Many primary care physicians will have had the experience of a patient with a functional or other ill-defined chronic disorder who finally reports considerable improvement after seeing a naturopathic physician. Some types of supplements long prescribed by naturopaths have now been studied and validated in clinical trials. Other features of naturopathic care may also be helpful to or resonate with patients. Naturopathic physicians may spend more time with their patients than their conventional medicine primary care peers, and their medical offices may provide for a less sterile and more pleasant and healing environment. Naturopaths will support and reinforce the world view of the patient who prefers dietary and herbal modalities to drugs in ways that allopathic physicians may not. Naturopaths will take time and effort to carefully review dietary and lifestyle patterns and may offer prescriptions in these areas at a level of detail that exceeds what is commonly provided by conventional primary care physicians. Naturopathic physicians have training and expertise in herbal medicines that allopathic physicians generally lack. Finally, in a clinical trial performed at the Kasier Permanente Center for Health Research in Portland, OR, assessing the impact of whole-system naturopathy on patients with temporomandibular joint dysfunction, multimodality naturopathic care provided for improvement in facial pain compared with conventional specialty temporomandibular joint dysfunction care.[94]

Although many patients can benefit from naturopathic care, conflicts exist between the naturopathic and conventional medicine paradigms and practice. The most frequently encountered example relates to evaluation and management of thyroid disorders. Naturopathic physicians will commonly recommend multiple hormone studies, including T3 and T4 levels, in settings where, from a primary care internal medicine perspective, the sensitive thyroid stimulating hormone (TSH) test is the only appropriate test. (T3, T4, and TSH are different types of thyroid-related hormones that circulate in the body).

The discrepancies can extend to patient management as well. Naturopaths will typically advise patients to supplement with combination T3-T4 preparations, such as desiccated thyroid. This contradicts conventional endocrine guidelines for T4 supplementation alone in the setting of hypothyroidism. The reasons underlying the conventional recommendation are: Desiccated thyroid preparations may provide inconsistent levels of thyroid hormone from one batch to the next. T3-containing preparations may also provide for more fluctuation, and a less steady state of thyroid hormone levels because of the rapid gastrointestinal absorption and the relatively short half-life of T3. In addition, blinded randomized controlled trial data have shown no benefit of combination T3-T4 preparations over T4 in terms of patients' symptoms and quality of life.[95] Nevertheless, patients understandably become confused when they are hearing one thing from the naturopathic physician and the opposite from the endocrinologist or primary care physician.

The main reason it is so hard for your naturopathic physician and your primary care physician to work together is because naturopathy defines not a modality, but rather an approach to the patient, or a system of care. Allopathic medicine is also a system, but the 2 systems offer perspectives and prescriptions that often contradict one another. Chinese medicine, too, is a system of care, but people have extracted and isolated acupuncture as a modality, that we can then compartmentalize, evaluate, and integrate, like any other procedure. Likewise for chiropractic care and spinal manipulation. In contrast, there is no such signature naturopathic procedure to sink our teeth into. What we are left with is 2 competing views of the world.

> Naturopathic and conventional medicine physicians sometimes disagree with one another, which creates confusion for the patient. The most common subject of disagreement is in the area of endocrine, or hormonal, disorders.

The bottom line is that many patients benefit from seeing a naturopathic physician, but sometimes naturopathy directly contradicts conventional care. When this occurs, the situation can be tricky for the patient to navigate, as well as frustrating for the physicians. Given the chronic shortage of primary care physicians, we can envision that naturopathic physicians, as a profession, could provide an important boost to primary care manpower. Achieving this on any scale will require more dialogue between the naturopathic and allopathic communities about how to bridge the gaps in paradigm and practice styles.

> If you are seeing both an allopathic physician and a naturopathic physician, consider suggesting that they communicate with one another. Please do not expect your primary care physician to order tests that have been suggested by the naturopathic physician. The primary care physician may not necessarily be able to order the tests, or may not agree that they are needed.

In the meantime, if you are seeing both an allopathic physician and a naturopathic physician, consider suggesting that they communicate with one another. On the other hand, many times patients will ask their primary care physician to order tests that have been suggested by the naturopathic physician so that the tests can be covered by the patient's health insurance policy. Such requests should be avoided because the primary care physician may not necessarily be able to order the tests, or may not agree that they are needed.

Homeopathy is another of the well-known systems of complementary medicine. The homeopathic practitioner treats "like with like." For example, suppose a patient presents with nausea. In allopathic medicine we would treat the patient with an anti-emetic, a medication that reduces nausea. In homeopathy, the approach would be the opposite. The homeopath identifies a substance that at full dose causes nausea, maximally dilutes it, and then treats the patient with this diluted remedy. In practice the situation is more complex because patients commonly present with a multitude of symptoms, and identifying the correct remedy for a patient's symptom pattern requires sophisticated analysis. Another system of complementary medicine called *anthroposophy*[96] includes homeopathic types of remedies and is commonly practiced in Europe.

Homeopathy is popular, and to a limited extent has been studied. Results of these studies show promise, but more high-quality research is needed.[97] Because they are so diluted, genuine homeopathic remedies can be considered safe.

Another popular system of integrative medicine is *functional medicine.* Functional medicine is "a personalized, systems-oriented model that empowers patients and practitioners to achieve the highest expression of health by working in collaboration to address the underlying causes of disease."[98] A growing number of medical physicians have sought training in and have begun integrating this approach. The functional medicine practitioner aims to treat chronic disease at its root cause using a systems-oriented perspective. The practice of functional medicine frequently involves a lot of laboratory testing. Many of these tests are unconventional or unorthodox from the allopathic medicine perspective. Treatment commonly includes the purchase of a significant number of nutritional or nutraceutical supplements.

The functional medicine movement has made a number of significant contributions. These practitioners have correctly identified that a more holistic paradigm is needed in medicine, and by training physicians and offering novel therapeutics to patients, have taken material steps to do something about it. Unlike those who have imported Asian paradigms into integrative medicine practices, the functional medicine community attempts to evolve a Western system of holistic care. This in principle makes a lot of sense. Finally, the functional medicine group has achieved substantial hegemony within integrative medicine in North America, and as such represents an important voice. However, as a movement, functional medicine is only a few decades old, with relatively little in the way of either history of use or rigorous outcomes data. Because many of the laboratory evaluations and treatment approaches within functional medicine seem alien to, or even at odds with, contemporary conventional medicine practice, we will need to stay tuned to see what kind of evidence base evolves, before it can be determined what kind of role functional medicine should play.

PART III. LET'S GET SPECIFIC

An overview of specific approaches tailored to particular health concerns

CHAPTER ELEVEN

MORE TO DIGEST

Practical guidelines for improving common digestive problems, including constipation, irritable bowel syndrome, food intolerances, and heartburn.

In Chapter Two, we explained that according to ayurveda, digestive issues represent a significant contributing cause in the pathogenesis of multiple chronic health disorders. Therefore, when a patient comes to our office with a chronic health problem, we almost always assume a digestive component and treat accordingly. At minimum, we emphasize the following points to nearly every patient presenting with a chronic health issue:

1. Have your main meal at midday!
2. Dinner should be light.
3. No snacking after dinner.

Remarkably, many symptoms, including gastrointestinal symptoms, significantly improve with these simple measures alone.

When patients report specific digestive complaints, we must always confirm that serious or life-threatening causes have been excluded. In our integrative medicine clinic, patients usually have already had a thorough evaluation by the time they are referred to us. Most commonly, the referring physician has already ordered the scans, endoscopies, blood work, and other needed tests, and these have already proved unrevealing. If such an evaluation has not been done, we perform a thorough assessment and schedule the patients for any tests that are indicated.

The treatment approach for digestive complaints from an ayurvedic vantage point depends on the specific symptom complex. We first ask patients about bowel habits and initially focus on correcting *constipation* if present. According to ayurveda, a normal bowel movement first thing every morning, without straining, signals proper gut function and health. Of course, many patients with constipation report hard stools, with the bowels moving only every two or three days. However, even if a patient comes to us and says, "My bowel movements are fine. I have a bowel movement first thing in the afternoon," we still consider this a constipation issue. Ideally, the patient should have a bowel movement immediately on awakening, every morning.

Constipation, when present, not only signals imbalanced digestive and physiologic function, but also contributes to multiple common health complaints. For example, recall that vata dosha governs movement. Each of the 3 doshas has 5 subdoshas. One of the subdoshas of vata called "apana vata" governs movement in the downward direction. According to ayurvedic theory, constipation causes blockage of apana vata. Such an obstruction can result in the reversal of the natural downward flow of energy toward the upward direction, which in turn can lead to headaches and other symptoms.

> **This is a cardinal principle in medicine: Whenever one suffers from constipation or has difficulty moving his bowels, serious diseases will beset him.**
> — Maimonides, Mishneh Torah, Hilchot De'ot 4:13

We commonly provide patients who report constipation with the following initial protocol. These guidelines include both daily and weekly routines for normalizing bowel function and improving symptoms.

Self-Care Protocol For Constipation

When you wake up, have a glass of warm water with a teaspoon of raw honey and a squirt (5-10 drops) of fresh lemon juice. Stir briskly to mix the honey in the water. This not only serves a cleansing function but also triggers a gastric-colic reflex resulting in a prompt bowel movement. Remember that the honey must be raw, and the water warm but not hot. (One should not add honey to boiling hot water because cooked honey is toxic). After drinking the warm honey-lemon water, consider taking a few minutes to sit on the commode to allow for a bowel movement to occur. Do this even if you do not have any sensation that a bowel movement is imminent. This practice helps train the physiology to get the bowels moving first thing every morning. If you don't have raw honey or lemon, just use warm water.

With breakfast, include a handful of soaked prunes or raisins. Soak these in a bowl with just enough water to cover the fruit overnight, then eat them with breakfast the next morning. Soaking in water renders the dried fruit much easier to digest. If you have a lot of pitta in your constitution, avoid the prunes and stick with the soaked raisins. Prunes can aggravate pitta dosha because of their sour taste.

Lunch should be the main meal of the day. We have earlier discussed this in great detail. See Chapter Three for some great menu options.

Dinner should be lighter.

Include a cup of cooked greens with lunch and/or dinner. Remember, this means a total of at least one cup of greens *after* they are cooked. We are talking about a lot of greens! Favor leafy green vegetables like spinach, chard, kale, bok choy, mustard greens, beet greens, and collard greens. Chop the greens before cooking and add a few drops of oil and spices as they cook. See Chapter Three for additional details.

At bedtime, take 2 g to 3 g of triphala with a little warm water. Triphala is a well-known ayurvedic mixture composed of three herbal ingredients. Triphala serves as a gastrointestinal tonic and has a mild laxative effect. You can find triphala at most health food stores, pharmacies, and other retail outlets that stock supplements. You also have the option of ordering the supplement online. Please reference the Resources section at the end of the book for some suggested suppliers. In any case, do your homework and be sure to purchase a quality product.

Try the "hot-water routine." Drink frequent sips of hot water throughout the day. We advise our patients to purchase a thermos, then fill the thermos with plain hot water that has been boiled in an uncovered pot for 5 minutes, and sip it throughout the day. If the weather is very hot or you are having hot flashes, let the water cool down a bit before sipping. Drinking water that has been boiled in an uncovered pot helps to balance all of the doshas.

Do a 24-hour liquid fast once a week: We advise patients to do a 24-hour liquid fast, from lunch to lunch, weekly. The patient eats a normal lunch, then takes nothing solid until lunch the next day. We are not requiring zero calories for 24 hours, just nothing solid. You can have juices, milk, purees, and so on, for both dinner and breakfast. For example, instead of solid foods for dinner, have a glass of warm milk, or cook up some vegetables and puree them in their cooking water in a sturdy glass blender. Likewise, for breakfast, have some tea, warm milk, or some fresh squeezed juice.

The above outlined protocol for improving constipation will provide excellent results for most people. If, however, you have not achieved the desired results after 4-6 weeks, you can also try the following tip. Fill up a *copper bowl or pitcher* with fresh water, place the vessel at your bedside, and drink the water early in the morning. Drink as much as you can. Several weeks of this practice can help the bowels to start functioning properly.

When patients report other gastrointestinal problems, we identify the specific digestive imbalance and treat accordingly. In particular, we determine whether the symptoms suggest a vata digestive imbalance, a pitta digestive imbalance, or a kapha digestive imbalance.

Symptoms of *vata digestive imbalance* commonly include gas, bloating, cramping, and constipation, and in many patients correlate with the allopathic diagnosis of *irritable bowel syndrome*. Irregular or frequently changing symptoms also suggest a vata type of digestive imbalance. Symptoms of pitta digestive imbalance commonly include hyperacidity and esophageal reflux. *Pitta digestive imbalance* can also lead to chronic loose stools. *Kapha digestive imbalance* will commonly present with heaviness of the abdomen, nausea, sticky bowel movements, and increased mucus.

In all of these situations we advise the guidelines for improving and maintaining proper digestion, as detailed in earlier chapters and summarized at the end of Chapter Four. In addition, we may offer some of the following specific recommendations.

For *vata digestive imbalance*, we advise a vata-balancing diet (see Chapter Five). Eating on a regular schedule is strongly emphasized. Food should be fresh, warm, and well-cooked. Include plenty of cooked greens in the diet. Add fresh spices such as chopped fresh ginger, cumin, mustard seeds, and asafetida, sautéed briefly in a little ghee or olive oil, to your vegetable or main course at lunch time. Avoid heavier foods including meats and cheeses, as well as deep-fried foods. Avoid cold or frozen foods. Reduce or avoid nut butters, fermented foods, and carbonated beverages.

Specific foods that can have a therapeutic effect for vata digestive imbalance include ghee, which enhances agni, as well as lassi. Favor cooked fruit, such as stewed apples, pears, raisins, dates, and figs, as well as other sweet fruits. We also recommend plenty of fiber in the diet, including cooked leafy greens, soaked or cooked nuts and seeds, and whole grains. Metamucil serves as a fiber supplement that can also be of benefit in this setting.

Ginger tea can have a positive therapeutic effect. Also, you can apply oil (sesame or castor) around the navel followed by hot water bottle application. A traditional ayurvedic herbal formula called Hingavashtak Churna can be effective for vata digestive imbalance. The appropriate dose is 2 g to 4 g with warm water before meals. (MAPI [see Resources] sells this mixture as MA 685.)

For *pitta digestive imbalance*, follow the pitta-balancing diet (see Chapter Five). Avoid foods that are hot and spicy, as well as foods that are too sour or salty. Patients must also avoid carbonated beverages, as well as eating too heavily at night. Patients must eliminate, or severely reduce, vinegar, alcohol, and red meat. We encourage stress management techniques (see Chapter Seven) and remind the patient to eat in a settled environment. Patients should avoid eating during meetings or under stressful circumstances. We instruct patients to favor sweet juicy fruits, including melons. Coconut is also very pitta pacifying.

Following are some traditional and home remedies for esophageal reflux, hyperacidity, and other pitta-related digestive symptoms.

- Therapeutic herbal tea:

  1 teaspoon coriander
  1 teaspoon fennel
  1 teaspoon cardamom

  Boil spices in 2 to 4 cups of hot water for 3 minutes. Strain, pour into a thermos, and sip warm throughout the day.
- Drink ¼ to ½ cup aloe vera juice after lunch and dinner.
- On an as-needed basis, sip a cup of warm milk with 2 teaspoons of either rose water or rose petal preserves.
- Chew cardamom seeds periodically throughout the day.
- Amalaki (Indian Gooseberry) is an excellent rasayna (tonic) herb for balancing pitta. An appropriate dose is 2 g of the whole fruit (without seeds) twice daily.
- Avipattikar churna is a traditional ayurvedic formula that is helpful for managing hyperacidity and pitta digestive imbalance. The recommended dose is 2 g to 4 g per day with milk or warm water after meals (MAPI sells this mixture as "herbal acibalance").

When patients follow these guidelines, we often have success with tapering down, or off, acid-reducing medications such as cimetidine, famotidine, omeprazole, and others. Tapering is best done in consultation with your physician. Our usual approach is to implement the dietary and herbal protocol, then after a month or so we attempt to halve the dose of the pharmaceutical. Then, if the patient is doing well after 2 to 4 weeks, we can further taper the medication, or sometimes discontinue it altogether.

Patients with *kapha digestion imbalance* often present with sluggish digestion, including feelings of heaviness and fatigue after eating. These patients often are overweight and have difficulty losing pounds despite low digestive capacity and food intake. For kapha digestive imbalance, we advise a kapha-balancing diet (see Chapter Five). The patient must avoid cold, heavy, sweet, and oily foods. Frequent sips of ginger tea can be helpful. We advise the patient to favor light, bitter, and pungent foods, with a minimum of oil. A vegetarian diet should be favored, at least for the evening meal. Patients must avoid "puffy" breads. Flatbreads are okay but should be toasted. We encourage patients to wake up early every morning (by 6 a.m.), and to get some exercise every day (see Chapter Six). The patient must avoid daytime napping. Spicy lassi (lassi with cumin and a little salt) after lunch is prescribed as well (see recipe in Chapter Four). "*Ginger pickle*" can also be helpful. To prepare this, take a few slices of fresh ginger, and place them in a small cup or bowl. Squeeze the juice from a lemon over the ginger, add a little salt, and let the ginger soak in the lemon for an hour or so. Have this before lunch. Trikatu Churna (1 part each ginger, pippali, and black pepper) is a traditional ayurvedic formula that can be helpful for this symptom complex; take 2 g to 4 g with warm water or honey after meals. Another procedure that can benefit patients with kapha digestive imbalance is "virechena," which is discussed in the next chapter.

Finally, what about food allergies? Patients commonly present to our clinic with this concern. Sometimes patients are in fact allergic to specific foods, but clinically significant food allergies are nowhere near as common as people think. Lots of tests to look for specific food allergies are often not helpful or needed. Food intolerances, in contrast, are quite common, and are generally caused by 1 of 2 factors. Either the patient suffers from weak agni (digestion) or the patient is favoring foods that are contraindicated for his or her particular constitutional type. The appropriate management consists of implementing dietary guidelines to improve digestion, and/or adherence to the relevant dosha-specific diet.

PATIENT TESTIMONIAL

"I wanted to share with you my experience with Kaiser Permanente and the Natural Medicine program in the hope that my situation may help others with similar conditions.

A quick history

I had a major surgery in 2007. After recovering from this surgery I had several symptoms I couldn't seem to get a handle on. My primary care doctor diagnosed me with anxiety, depression, IBS, migraine, and insomnia. For 7 years I tried to find answers and treatment for these vague conditions with limited success.

Finally, earlier this year, my husband recommended I see his primary care physician, who is the lead in Natural Medicine. I switched doctors, went to your Natural Medicine class, and saw you for one appointment.

Within a few days of following your recommendations, my IBS symptoms, migraines, and anxiety/depression were greatly alleviated. Today, just a few weeks following my appointment with you, I'm feeling much improved, and feel no need for further medical intervention.

What this means is this—within 1 month I have a handle on 7 years of symptoms that had me baffled.

My well-intentioned Kaiser doctors prescribed Zoloft, Celexa, Trazodone, Ativan, Miralax, and Metamucil (a few others too for migraines but I can't remember the names), but no one ever mentioned nutrition or lifestyle changes. I know it is important to rule out medical conditions, so the myriad of labs and tests, including the colonoscopy I was given were important but ultimately unnecessary.

For a specific example: The GI doctor I was given met with me twice by phone only, and on both occasions told me to just keep taking Miralax, as much as I needed. I told him I was worried as I was up to 4 to 7 doses of it a day, and still not getting very good results. He told me I can keep taking more, and to add Metamucil too).

Since the cost of health care is a real and pressing issue, I wanted to communicate my experience so that other doctors might at the very least refer their patients to the Natural Medicine clinic or the class that you teach.

Above all I want to thank you, as I feel so much better … ."

CHAPTER TWELVE

MANAGING WITH CHRONIC PAIN

Ideas and tips for improving pain and function that put you in control of your health.

Patients commonly present to both primary care and complementary medicine clinicians with pain-related conditions. Although management can be challenging, fortunately we can offer many compelling treatments. As a rule, we recommend not only passive but also active interventions, because patients who actively involve themselves in managing their condition achieve the best improvements in function and reductions in pain. The importance of this last point cannot be overemphasized.

Although we cannot always completely resolve a patient's chronic pain, we offer strategies and advice to bring the situation under control. We work with the patient to implement a range of tools that maximize the patient's ability to enjoy hobbies, work productively, and to live a quality life.

Medications can help provide relief from chronic pain, but this is only part of the story. Medications alone generally don't solve the problem. In addition, pain medications can cause a lot of side effects. Anti-inflammatory pain killers can lead to stomach irritation and kidney problems. Opioid pain killers often cause constipation, mental dullness and confusion, fatigue, and other problems, and can lead to addiction. We set a goal of reducing medications to the minimum possible amount.

> **As to diseases, make a habit of two things—to help, or at least to do no harm.**
> — Hippocrates, Epidemics

In Chapter Two, we learned how and why digestive challenges contribute to problems like chronic pain. According to ayurveda, weak digestion can lead to accumulation of ama (the toxic byproduct of improper digestion). This ama then deposits in the joints, muscles, and other connective tissues, causing pain, stiffness, and fatigue. One of the main approaches we adopt in managing chronic pain is the reduction and elimination of ama. We review the dietary guidelines detailed in Chapters Two through Four with each patient, and we emphasize the appropriate dosha-specific menu for managing digestive symptoms, as detailed in Chapter Five. In addition, for many patients presenting with chronic pain, we will advise ama pachana, which is a set of recommendations geared toward detoxification, i.e., removal of ama. We would not expect an individual patient to do ALL of the things listed below. Rather, we provide a range of options and work with each patient to select the suitable, individualized subset.

Self-Care Procedures For Detoxification (Ama Pachana)

1. Be sure to use plenty of the following spices with your cooking: ginger, cumin, black pepper, fennel, hing, basil, mustard seeds.
2. Eat your main meal at midday! Dinner should be light, i.e., soup with toasted flatbread or cooked cereal with warm milk.
3. No snacking after dinner!
4. Ginger pickle: As described in Chapter Eleven (in the section on managing kapha digestive imbalance). Avoid if there is hyperaciditiy or pitta imbalance.
5. First thing in the morning, have a glass of warm water with a teaspoon of raw honey and a squirt of lemon.
6. "Hot-water routine": This means frequent sips of hot water throughout the day.
7. 24-hour liquid fast once a week: This provides a great tool for resetting agni and reducing ama (see Chapter Eleven, section on management of constipation).

Scientific data support the traditional ayurvedic recommendation of fasting as an approach for managing chronic pain. Fasting and caloric restriction have been shown to provide marked anti-inflammatory and mood-enhancing effects.[99] In one study, fasting followed by a vegetarian diet led to significant reductions in pain and joint inflammation for patients with rheumatoid arthritis.[100]

8. Virechana: Home purgation protocol *(Note: This procedure should be done only under the supervision of a physician. Patients with severe vata imbalance, very weak agni, and patients with gallstones should not do virechana.)*

Virechana refers to a home purgation protocol that can be done as often as once a month, but not more frequently. Virechana promotes elimination of ama, as well as removal of excess pitta dosha.

Fourteen-day ginger program	
Day	# of slices of ginger
1	1
2	2
3	3
4	4
5	5
6	6
7	7
8	7
9	6
10	5
11	4
12	3
13	2
14	1

The entire protocol takes 4 days. Patients should stick with a very light diet during this period. The first 3 days of the protocol provide for "oleation." On day 1, take 4 teaspoons of melted ghee on an empty stomach. Take no other food or beverage except for warm water for 2 to 3 hours, or until hunger returns. On day 2, repeat the procedure using 6 teaspoons of ghee, and on day 3 take 8 teaspoons. Although a light diet must be maintained, it is okay to work and to go about your normal activities during the 3 days of oleation.

On day 4 you will do the purgation (virechana) procedure. This must be a day of rest, without going to work. To do the virechana, you need 3 to 8 teaspoons of castor oil, a glass, some water, and an orange. If you have a tendency toward diarrhea, use a lower dose of castor oil (closer to 3 teaspoons), but if you have tendency toward constipation, use a higher dose (closer to 8 teaspoons). Again, only do this on a morning when you will be able to rest. Pour the castor oil into a glass, squeeze in the juice from half an orange, dilute with water, and drink. Then, bite into the other half of the orange and chew vigorously. We expect 4 to 5 loose bowel movements during the next few hours. Fast, except for sips of hot water, until the effect has worn off. You presumably will be able to have a light lunch, provided that you start off early in the morning.

As an alternative to the above protocol, you can include in your diet a teaspoon of castor oil mixed with food daily for 4 to 6 weeks. When the castor oil is taken this way, no preliminary oleation is required, so this could be a preferred approach for someone who cannot tolerate the larger amount of ghee, or if taking extra ghee is contraindicated (for example, if there is a problem with heart disease or high cholesterol).

9. Digestive decoction recipe: *(We advise against using this decoction if there is a pitta imbalance, such as symptoms of frequent heartburn, or reflux.)* Boil 1 quart of water with 1 teaspoon cumin seeds, 1 teaspoon coriander seeds, 1 teaspoon fresh grated ginger, ½ teaspoon fresh lemon juice, and 2 pinches of black pepper. You may add 1 teaspoon of raw sugar to taste if desired, as well as 2 pinches of black salt if it is available. Place in a thermos and sip throughout the day (not in the evening). This decoction can be used in place of the plain hot water suggested as part of the hot water routine.
10. Ginger 14-day program: *(Do not do this ginger protocol if you have frequent heartburn or other symptoms of gastric hyperacidity.)* On day 1, chew 1 slice of fresh ginger first thing in the morning. Breakfast should be very light, or skipped. Each subsequent day, add an additional slice of ginger for a total of 7 days. On day 8, repeat with 7 slices of

ginger and taper 1 slice less per day until day 14, when you have only 1 slice again.

11. Sweating is good for reducing ama. This can be accomplished by periodically visiting the sauna.

These guidelines for ama reduction can help not only patients with chronic pain, but also those with any ama-related pattern of symptoms, including depression, low energy, and fatigue.

When a patient suffering from an ama-related condition does not respond to the home care measures outlined above, the patient may benefit from "*panchakarma.*"

Panchakarma provides a series of intensive detoxification treatments done under close supervision of an ayurvedic physician. Only trained and qualified personnel can provide these treatments, which are frequently done in a spa or residential setting. The modalities provided as part of panchakarma include a special diet, massage with herbalized oils, as well as elimination therapies, including both virechena and the administration of herbalized enemas. Several reputable centers in North America provide these treatments. We have included some recommended facilities in the Resources section at the end of the book, and when appropriate, we advise our patients to consider them. Data support the traditional claim that panchakarma detoxifies the physiology. For example, scientific studies have shown an association between the administration of panchakarma procedures and reductions in fat soluble toxicants[101] and lipid peroxide levels.[102]

In addition to medication management and ama pachana, patients with chronic pain should exercise as much as possible.

> **Whoever is idle and does not exercise, or does not move his bowels when he has the need, or is constipated, even if he eats the proper foods and takes care to follow the rules of medicine, will be full of pain for all his days and his strength will fade away.**
> — Maimonides, *Mishneh Torah, Hilchot De'ot* 4:15.

In the setting of chronic pain, regular exercise can both improve function and reduce pain intensity.[103,104] The patient can choose walking, going to the gym, lifting weights, water aerobics, or whatever s/he finds enjoyable and sustainable. Importantly, finding a routine you enjoy will lead to a sustainable program. One should avoid falling into the practice of exercising intensely for a few weeks and then just dropping it. The patient should focus on developing a routine that is practical and sustainable over time. Patients can also consider yoga as part of an exercise regimen in managing pain (see Chapter Seven).

We also re-emphasize the central importance of daily routine (See Chapter Six). Getting to bed on time, waking up early in the morning, and exercising in the morning on a regular basis will all contribute to progress in achieving improvements in pain and energy levels. Patients should avoid excess traveling, tobacco, drugs, and alcohol. Mind-body and stress-reduction techniques (see Chapter Seven) also make a valuable contribution to self-care.

We additionally recommend to many patients a fabulous self-care procedure called abhyanga. This is a daily oil massage self-administered by the patient immediately before taking a bath or shower. The best oil to use for most patients is sesame oil (see Sidebar: Sesame Oil). Some patients with too much pitta will not tolerate sesame oil on the skin due to its heating qualities. In these instances, one can substitute with coconut oil or olive oil.

SESAME OIL

According to ayurveda, sesame ranks among the best oils for therapeutic massage. Sesame oil balances all three doshas, and achieves good penetration of the skin.[15] Scientists have shown that sesame oil has anticarcinogenic,[105] antioxidant,[106] and anti-inflammatory[107] properties. In the study by Monteiro and colleagues,[107] sesame oil was administered orally to experimental mice and rats who were then exposed to various noxious stimulae. Compared with animals who were fed just salt water, those receiving sesame oil orally took longer to react to high-heat application to their paws and showed less swelling of the paws after injection of an irritant. In another experiment,[108] the investigators randomly assigned 150 people with extremity trauma to receive either topical sesame oil application plus usual care or usual care alone. Those receiving the sesame oil topical application showed reductions in pain severity and pain medication use compared with the control group.

In addition to serving as an excellent therapeutic massage oil, sesame oil can play a role in the maintenance of the health of the teeth, gums, and nasal passages. Ayurveda prescribes that a sesame oil mouthwash be performed daily for the purpose of maintaining the health of the teeth and gums. You can do this procedure first thing in the morning. Place 1 to 2 tablespoons of sesame oil in your mouth. Swish the oil around in your mouth for about 2 minutes, then gargle for 15 seconds, and spit out the sesame oil in a cup. (It's best to not spit oil down the drain because this can eventually clog the drain. The oil can later be disposed of in the garbage.) Next,` place some sesame oil on your fingertip and massage the gum line for about a minute. Finally, rinse with warm water. Scientists have documented the beneficial effect of sesame oil mouthwash on reducing bacterial colony counts,[109] and on other measures of oral hygiene, in several clinical trials.[110]

A procedure called "nasya" can help promote the health of the nasal passages and sinuses. Place a few drops of sesame oil in the palm of your hand. Dip your index finger into the oil, then apply to the inside of one nostril, and inhale. Repeat on the other side. You can do nasya daily.

Before performing the oil massage, the sesame oil should be "cured." To accomplish this, pour the oil into a saucepan and place it on your stovetop on low-medium heat. After a few minutes, place a drop of water into the oil. When the drop of water "sizzles," then that batch of oil has been successfully cured. Oil is flammable, so be sure to heat it up gradually, on lower heat as opposed to high heat, and do not leave the heating oil unattended. Note that if you are using coconut or olive oil instead of sesame oil, they do not need to be cured. After curing the oil, using a funnel or a steady hand, you can pour it into smaller plastic squirt-top bottles for ease of use.

You will then perform the oil massage just before your warm bath or shower. Bathing after the oil massage actually enhances the body's deep absorption of the oil. Oil application after bathing is felt not to have such a positive effect. Morning is the best time, but later in the day or in the evening is also okay. Start with your head and work your way down. If you are washing your hair you will begin with the scalp, otherwise skip the scalp and begin with the face. Apply some oil to the palm of your hand and massage it into your scalp. Do the same with the face, and then the back of the neck. Extra attention should be paid to massage the oil into the temples. When you apply oil to the arms, use the palm of your hand and massage the oil around in a circle over the joints, and up and down over the long bones. Do not forget to include the hands and fingers. Apply the oil to the chest, then the abdomen, in a circular, clockwise direction. You should apply oil to the upper and lower parts of your back as best as you can reach. Next, approach the legs in the same way as the arms. Apply the oil to the joints in a circular motion, while massaging up and down over the long bones, beginning at the hip and working your way down. Finally, be certain to focus a little extra attention on massaging the oil into the soles of the feet.

After completing this oil massage you can sit for a few minutes and then step into the shower. Ideally you should allot about 15 to 20 minutes to doing the oil massage, but if you are pressed for time you can do the entire abhyanga in just 7 to 10 minutes. You can also substitute an abbreviated "short-abhyanga," if necessary. This involves performing the massage on only the temples and the soles of the feet and takes just a couple of minutes.

To learn more about how to do the abhyanga oil massage, you can watch any of several videos available on YouTube, including: www.youtube.com/watch?v=nMOGvuNtxvY; www.youtube.com/watch?v=_HQLsfZh5js.

Done regularly, this oil massage will help reduce and prevent chronic musculoskeletal pain. The oil massage provides multiple other health benefits as well, including relaxation of the nervous system and improvement of the luster of the skin.

A few practical tips warrant mention. Reserve a specific set of towels for drying off after you have done your oil massage and shower. The oil will penetrate the towels, and after a while can be hard to wash out. You don't want to ruin all of your towels. Also, be mindful of keeping the floor of the shower clean to avoid slipping.

Ideally, you should add the oil massage to your routine on a daily basis. Wake up early, meditate, then exercise. After you exercise, do your abhyanga and shower. At mid-day, have a good lunch. Meditate late in the afternoon, and be certain to get to bed by 10 p.m. Next day, repeat, and so on. There you have it, the *picture of health!*

Many herbs and supplements help with the management of chronic pain. These supplements are effective for many people, and generally have fewer dangerous effects compared with nonsteroidal anti-inflammatory medications (like ibuprofen or naproxen) or opioids (like morphine or hydrocodone). Individual supplements that can help reduce pain include turmeric, boswellia, and glucosamine sulfate. Refer to Chapter Eight for further information and dosing instructions. Remember that your physician or practitioner may also recommend a multi-ingredient herbal formula specific to your personal constitutional type or individual situation.

We often advise our patients with chronic pain to take lessons in the Alexander Technique. This technique offers an approach to the health of the mind and body with an emphasis on releasing counterproductive habits, especially those related to posture and the spine. Studies have shown that lessons in the Alexander Technique result in improvements for patients with chronic spine-related pain.[111] You can learn more, and find a local Alexander Technique teacher, through the American Society for the Alexander Technique (www.amsatonline.org). The Feldenkrais method provides another potentially effective option for patients.[112] Not only physical therapy, but also acupuncture, chiropractic care, and massage therapy can all effectively contribute to pain management, as reviewed in Chapter Nine.

The approach to *chronic headaches* will depend on the overall pattern of symptoms described by the patient. In general, tension headaches represent a vata imbalance, migraine headaches represent a pitta imbalance, whereas sinus headaches represent kapha imbalance. We prescribe the appropriate dietary (see Chapter Five), behavioral, and herbal regimen according to the primary doshic imbalance. Both constipation (see

Chapter Eleven) and menstrual irregularities (see Chapter Fifteen) can indirectly cause headaches through blockage of the apana vata subdosha, and need to be corrected when present. An herbal supplement called MigreLief is effective for preventing migraine headaches (see Chapter Eight). In addition, amla berry (Indian gooseberry) can also be useful for headache management. Two grams of the whole fruit (without seeds) twice daily is an appropriate dose.

In summary, patients with chronic pain can choose from a range of holistic remedies and tools to match their needs, preferences, and lifestyles. These self-care approaches can empower the patient to reduce pain, improve function, and take control of his/her health.

Patients with chronic pain often suffer from *depression* and/or *anxiety* as well, and the patient and physician should not overlook addressing these issues. Patients suffering from *depression* must emphasize engaging in purposeful activities and exercising adequately. Thirty to 60 minutes of vigorous daily physical exercise is a must. We emphasize a regular routine with an early bedtime, and recommend a morning walk in the rising sun. Patients with depression benefit from being with friends, staying involved socially, and playing with children. We advise depressed patients to take fresh warm meals, and to avoid alcohol and tamasic foods, including red meat, canned foods, cold foods, frozen and junk foods, excessive sweets, and leftovers. Several supplements can help with depression, including St. John's Wort and Ashwagandha (see Chapter Eight). The combination of the supplements "Blissful Joy" (1 tablet twice daily) and "Mind Plus" syrup (1 to 2 teaspoons twice daily), available through MAPI (www.mapi.com) provides an excellent effect for many people.

For patients suffering from anxiety, meditation plays an especially critical role (see Chapter Seven). In terms of diet, patients must eat warm, cooked meals on a regular schedule, and avoid caffeinated beverages. We encourage patients with anxiety to engage in uplifting physical activity, including gardening and yard work. The daily oil massage with sesame oil provides important benefit. We advise patients to maintain a regular routine, including early bedtime by 10 p.m. and 30 minutes of walking daily, best done in the morning sun (see Chapter Six). Supplements that may be of benefit include bacopa (see Chapter Eight). Many of our patients improve using the combination of the supplements "Worry Free" tablets (1 tablet twice daily) and "Mind Plus" syrup (1 to 2 teaspoons twice daily), available through MAPI. Aromatherapy with lavender[113] or other essential aroma oils can also be effective.

Case Study

"JS" is a 61-year-old woman who came to our clinic seeking help with symptoms of chronic musculoskeletal pain, including back pain and fibromyalgia. Her symptoms were so severe that she was requiring high doses of opioid pain medications on a daily basis to try to control her pain. When she first came to our clinic she was taking methadone in doses of 40 mg a day. She was very motivated and wanted to reduce her use of the medication and to improve her symptoms using lifestyle and natural approaches.

We provided her with guidelines for improving digestion and for maintaining a proper daily routine. She was instructed regarding a healthy diet and advised to exercise on a regular basis. We also advised her to learn and use a stress-reduction technique.

The patient worked to improve her lifestyle and diet, quit smoking, and enrolled in a course to learn the Transcendental Meditation technique. She continues to focus on improving her diet and losing weight, and still meditates on a regular basis. Over a period of 4 years she has succeeded in reducing her methadone dose from 40 mg per day to 12.5 mg per day.

CHAPTER THIRTEEN

TO STATIN OR NOT TO STATIN?

Holistic approaches to help with high blood pressure, obesity, diabetes, and cardiovascular disease, including how to make the smartest choice about statin medication.

Although medications play an important role in managing high blood pressure, we in addition emphasize holistic and self-care approaches as much as is practical. Diet and exercise alone can affect high blood pressure to a meaningful degree. We recommend that patients with high blood pressure exercise for at least 30 minutes, at least 6 days a week. Specific dietary measures include limiting salt intake, while increasing fresh fruits and fresh-cooked vegetables.

According to a position paper published by the American Heart Association,[43] 3 complementary and integrative medicine interventions have been found effective and are appropriate to recommend for patients with high blood pressure. These include the Transcendental Meditation (TM) program, the "resperate" device, and biofeedback. Regular practice of the TM technique lowers blood pressure about as effectively as taking a single blood pressure medication. We reviewed this technique in detail in Chapter Seven. "Resperate" is a device that guides a relaxation exercise focused on slowing the patient's breathing. Use of the device results in lower blood pressure. You can get information and purchase the device online at www.resperate.com. Biofeedback techniques use electronic monitoring of blood pressure and other physiologic parameters to help the patient devise mental and behavioral strategies for reducing high blood pressure. For patients with high blood pressure who want to use a scientifically proven nonpharmacologic approach, these 3 approaches can help.

Two-thirds of adults in the US are either obese or overweight. Many patients present to our clinic requesting help with weight management. Although the reasons for the obesity epidemic are multiple and complex, ayurveda provides a useful analysis that can help some patients better understand and more effectively address the situation. People in our society experience lots of stress and are always on the go. Running around, always trying to do too much, aggravates vata dosha. Then, to balance the aggravated vata, people naturally crave vata-pacifying foods. Which type of foods balance vata? Those that are heavy, oily, salty, and sweet! When vata dosha is out of balance, eating such foods makes us feel better, but only up to a certain point. If the causative lifestyle factors aren't corrected, the vata imbalance persists, and we continue to crave the heavy oily salty and sweet food. Such a diet inevitably leads to kapha imbalance, with weight gain.

Understanding and correcting a vata-aggravating lifestyle goes a long way toward helping with weight loss. Most importantly, people need to reduce and to effectively manage stress (see Chapter Seven), and to stick with a good daily routine (see Chapter Six). In the end, the effective approach to losing weight requires reducing caloric intake along with increasing exercise. In other words, the patient must achieve a negative caloric balance. Our goal, then, is to help the patient devise an individualized strategy to accomplish this. We generally do not emphasize supplements for weight management because the supplements available for this purpose are for the most part either ineffective or dangerous. A good initial step for the patient is to simply reduce portion sizes by 15% to 20%. You can continue eating the diet you are accustomed to, but less food. Combine this with regular exercise, at least 180 minutes/week (minimum 30 minutes a day, 6 days a week). Maintaining a simple program like this can achieve weight loss of a few pounds a month. We recommend a slow-steady approach of this type as opposed to dramatic weight loss. It is better to take the weight off slowly and to keep it off than to lose a bunch of weight only to regain that much and more in the following months. Think about weight loss as a transition to a healthier lifestyle for the long haul.

Any program that provides you with monitoring, positive reinforcement, and peer support will be helpful. The commercial weight loss programs, like Weight Watchers, often provide benefit in this regard. We don't feel that buying supplements and food from programs is what's needed; instead, it's the peer support that some programs offer that can be helpful. We encourage patients to weigh themselves daily and to maintain a food diary of some sort. Regularly monitoring your weight and food intake will help you to achieve, and then to maintain, your weight loss goals.

Patients with type 2 diabetes frequently require medications to optimally manage their condition. However, diet, exercise, weight loss, stress reduction, and sometimes supplements also play an important role.[114] Stress aggravates blood sugar problems, and studies have shown that meditation practices can help improve blood sugar control and reduce cardiovascular risk. In one randomized trial,[115] patients with coronary artery disease who learned to meditate showed reductions in both blood pressure and insulin resistance. Another cross-sectional study[116] showed that those who engaged in mind-body practices had significantly lower body mass indices, triglyceride levels, and fasting blood sugar levels, as well as a lower incidence of metabolic syndrome.

People with diabetes commonly use a number of popular supplements. Studies have shown *cinnamon* to be helpful in decreasing levels of fasting blood sugar, total cholesterol, LDL cholesterol, and triglyceride levels.[117] People use cassia cinnamon in doses of 120 mg to 6 g daily. *Fenugreek,* likewise, can lower blood sugar for patients with diabetes.[118] Typical dosing ranges from 5 g to 50 g/day of the powdered seed. *Bitter gourd* is a melon traditionally used to help lower blood sugars, and there, likewise, exists some evidence in the scientific literature to support this.[114] People commonly take 2 to 3 ounces of the juice once daily. The melon and the juice can be found in Indian and Asian food stores. Finally, chromium is a mineral found in some foods that can be effective for improving control of blood sugar in patients with diabetes.[119] Patients typically use 200 mcg to 1000 mcg daily.

In general, for patients with type 2 diabetes, these supplements can help, and alongside diet, exercise, medications, and stress reduction, can play a role in improving blood sugar control. As an alternative to purchasing a supplement, patients can also opt to include plenty of cinnamon and fenugreek as spices in the diet.

The ayurvedic diet for type 2 diabetes emphasizes small legumes, light grains, plenty of fresh-cooked vegetables, and low-fat dairy products, along with avoidance of sweets and excess carbohydrates. Studies have shown that consumption of a vegetarian diet reduces the risk of diabetes[120] and can improve control of blood sugar in patients with diabetes.[121]

The following ayurvedic dietary guidelines specific to the diabetic patient are adapted from our clinical trial protocol:[7]

General Ayurvedic Guidelines For The Diabetic Patient

1. Ideally, lunch should be the main meal of the day. Dinner should be lighter. This is because the body's digestive power is stronger at lunchtime.
2. Food should be fresh and warm. Leftovers, packaged foods, processed foods, and fast foods should be avoided. Cold foods and drinks should also be avoided.
3. Except for those with strong digestive capacity, raw vegetables should be avoided. Cooked vegetables are to be favored because they are more digestible. If taken, salads should be eaten at the beginning of the lunch meal only.

4. Aged, fermented, smoked, and pickled foods should be avoided.
5. Sugars should be avoided.
6. Honey should be avoided.
7. "Contrary" foods should be avoided. Examples of contrary foods are: a) milk together with sour foods, salty foods, spicy foods, or bitter foods, and vegetables; milk should also not be mixed with juices or citrus fruits; and b) hot and cold foods taken together at the same time.
8. Milk should be brought just to boiling with a pinch of turmeric before drinking it. It may subsequently be allowed to cool to room temperature before drinking, but should never be taken cold.
9. Yogurt and cheese should be avoided at night. If you have yogurt at lunch, it should be in diluted form, with 1 part yogurt mixed with 3 parts water. If you have cheese at lunch, it should be fresh, as opposed to aged.
10. Flatbreads like tortillas, chapatis, and pita breads are preferable to leavened, yeasted breads. If yeasted bread is taken, it should be toasted, and a little bit of oil (like clarified butter or olive oil) applied.
11. Staple breakfast foods include: cooked cereal, almonds (it is best to soak them and remove the skin before eating), and flatbreads.
12. Staple lunch foods include the following:
    a) Small legumes
       Split mung dal, other dals (e.g., channa dal), lentils, split peas, tofu, lima beans, nuts and seeds (nuts and seeds should be soaked in water or cooked).
       Large beans (such as kidney beans, black beans, and Mexican beans) should be taken less frequently.
    b) Grains
       Wheat (e.g., bulgur wheat, buckwheat, pasta), couscous, millet, quinoa, rye, amaranth, barley, polenta, kamut, spelt.
    c) Cooked vegetables.
    d) Toasted flatbreads like pita bread, tortillas, or chapatis (or toasted regular wheat bread).
    e) Lassi (diluted yogurt drink, salty) (see Chapter Four for recipe).
13. Supper will be similar to lunch, but take less quantity and favor lighter, more easily digestible foods such as light grains (couscous, millet, quinoa, corn, rye, bulgur wheat,

amaranth, barley), as opposed to heavy grains (rice, pasta).

14. For snacks during late afternoons, favor milk, or herbal tea, and toast.
15. At bedtime, boiled milk may be taken with a pinch of turmeric, cardamom, and saffron. Herbal tea may also be taken.
16. Meals should always be taken in a settled, calm atmosphere. Reading or watching television should be avoided during meals. Enough time should be allowed for meals so as to avoid feeling rushed. A few minutes of relaxation should be taken at the end of each meal.
17. One should eat warm, unctuous food in the proper quantity. Warm food tastes good, stimulates the digestive fire, gets digested quickly, and reduces flatus and mucous. Eating the proper quantity promotes lifespan and balanced excretory functions, and allows for digestion without discomfort. You should not eat again until the previously consumed meal has been digested. Nonantagonistic foods should be eaten, in a favorable place, with favorable accessories. Do not eat too quickly or too slowly. You should eat without much talking or laughing but with full concentration after due consideration to the self.
18. Food should always be pleasing to the senses.

Specific Meal Plans For The Diabetic Patient

Breakfast (7:30 to 8:30 a.m.)

1. Three to 5 tablespoons of hot cereal (crushed or broken grains), cooked with either water or skim or 1% or 2% milk. Add 2 to 3 teaspoons of soaked walnuts, pecans, sunflower seeds, pumpkin seeds, cracked hazelnuts, flax seeds, or sliced almonds. You may alternatively add 1 to 2 teaspoons of wheat germ.

   Examples of grains or cereals to use: 7 grain, bulgur wheat, quinoa, oatmeal, barley, rye, millet, spelt, kamut, and polenta. Ideally, grains should be pan roasted before cooking.

Other breakfast options could include:

2. Flatbreads such as tortillas or pita breads, slightly toasted. You can apply a small amount of either sesame, olive, or sunflower oil and eat with some steamed, chopped leafy greens or sprouts along with 2 teaspoons to 3 teaspoons of the above-mentioned nuts and seeds.
3. Flatbreads with veggie spread or pesto (without cheese).
4. Bean burrito with some steamed chopped vegetables.

Lunch (12:30 to 1:00 p.m.)

1. Toasted flatbreads (2 to 3 small pieces) and light grains (½ to 1 cup). Examples of appropriate grains include bulgur, barley, quinoa, millet, rye, polenta, kamut, spelt, and amarynth. If you like pasta, eat whole wheat, quinoa, or buckwheat pasta, and only once or twice a week. There should be more vegetables than pasta on the plate.
2. The number of cups of cooked vegetables you eat for lunch should correlate with the number of pieces of flatbread. One cup of cooked vegetables should be eaten per each piece of flatbread

   Favor the following vegetables:

   Green beans, fava beans, snow peas, green peas, artichoke, eggplant, plantain, brussel sprouts, bitter gourd, broccoli, cabbage, cauliflower, chayote squash, leeks, zucchini, celery, endive, tender asparagus, tender daikon (white) radish with small amount of green pepper.
3. In addition to the above vegetables, you should also include some cooked leafy greens at lunch: ½ to 1 cup chopped and steamed or pureed with some fresh spices like cilantro, basil, fresh ginger, mint, oregano, or parsley. Favor the following leafy greens: chard, kale, bokchoy, broccoli raab (rapini), chicory, escarole, arugula, watercress, dandelions, collard greens, fenugreek sprouts, Chinese cabbage, beet greens, mustard greens.
4. One cup well-cooked lentils, small beans, or split peas, with some fresh spices.
5. Two to 3 teaspoons soaked nuts or seeds (above mentioned with breakfast) taken separately or added to vegetables.
6. The ideal diet is a lactovegetarian diet. Nonvegetarians should favor light meats, such as fish and poultry, as opposed to red meats. Meats are better taken at lunch than at dinner.
7. Lassi (yogurt drink): 1 part yogurt, 3 parts water mix with ¼ teaspoon Turmeric.
8. Dessert is not recommended. (Some homemade cookies without sugar would be okay).

Afternoon snack (3:30 to 4:30 p.m.)

Choose one of the following:

1. Toast (flatbreads) with some oil, veggie spread, or pesto.
2. Rice cakes.
3. Corn chips (blue corn).
4. Popcorn without much grease.

5. Veggie burger (preferably homemade).
6. Bean burrito.

Dinner (6:00 to 7:00 p.m.)

1. Reduce or avoid grains. If taken, only light grains (see above) in a quantity of ½ to 1 cup should be taken.
2. Flatbreads, 2 to 3 pieces, with cooked vegetables, 2 to 3 cups.
3. Cooked leafy greens (½ to 1 cup after steamed), chopped and steamed, slightly spiced, and with a little olive oil.
4. One bowl of lentils, small beans, or spilt peas, with some fresh grated ginger or cilantro and some chopped vegetables.

Patients with coronary artery disease benefit from diet, exercise, weight loss, and stress reduction. Meditation practice has been shown to reverse atherosclerosis in patients with high blood pressure[122] and to improve performance on exercise testing in patients with coronary artery disease.[123] Lowering cholesterol levels can reduce your risk of heart disease and stroke, and the best way for most people to lower cholesterol is through lifestyle modification, including a proper diet and plenty of exercise. Note that consumption of a vegetarian diet (see Chapters Two to Five) has been found to be associated with lower levels of cholesterol and blood pressure, and with improvements in other markers of cardiovascular health.[124]

Patients seeking to lower their cholesterol commonly use a number of supplements. Red yeast rice is a supplement that has been shown to be effective in lowering cholesterol levels.[125] Red yeast rice contains several chemical constituents that are similar to statin drugs, and the concentration of these compounds can vary considerably from one brand of red yeast rice product to the next. *Guggul* is a plant-based resin that has been used to help improve high cholesterol; however, the evidence regarding its effectiveness is mixed.[126,127]

In addition to diet, exercise, and stress reduction, medications play an important role in the care of many patients with cardiovascular disease. We hear a lot about statin drugs (like lovastatin, simvastatin, pravastatin, and so on) from physicians, friends, and in the press. Indeed, physicians recommend statin drugs to nearly all patients with coronary artery disease, stroke history, or diabetes, and to many other patients as well. Yet many people remain skeptical about using statins, usually because of concerns about possible short- and long-term side effects. What is the underlying rationale behind the recommendation to use statin drugs? Is taking these medications really worth it?

Taking a statin drug reduces one's risk of heart attack and stroke. Specifically, taking a modest dose of a statin drug reduces your risk of having a heart attack or stroke over the next 10 years by about 20%, whereas taking a high dose of a statin drug reduces 10-year risk by about 40%. This is a huge risk reduction, and from these statistics it sounds like the decision in favor of taking the medications may be a no-brainer.

This is in fact what many people think, but before we jump to that conclusion, we first must further explore this idea of "risk reduction." Biomedical literature distinguishes between 2 different types of risk reduction: "relative" risk reduction and "absolute" risk reduction. To help us understand the difference and why it is important, consider the example of a patient who has a 10-year risk of heart attack or stroke of 14%. This 10-year risk can be calculated by a formula on the basis of age, gender, blood pressure, cholesterol values, blood sugar, and smoking status. The figure below, adopted from the Kaiser Permanente Northwest statin shared decision-making tool, helps us to understand what benefit such a patient may receive from taking a statin drug:

Based on your age and risk factors, you have a **14% chance** of having a heart attack or stroke in the next 10 years.
NO MEDICATION
86 out of 100 people will not have a heart attack or stroke.
14 out of 100 people will have a heart attack or stroke.
MODERATE DOSE STATIN
86 out of 100 people will not have a heart attack or stroke.
11 out of 100 people will have a heart attack or stroke.
3 out of 100 people will be saved from having a heart attack or stroke.
HIGH DOSE STATIN
86 out of 100 people will not have a heart attack or stroke.
8 out of 100 people will have a heart attack or stroke.
6 out of 100 people will be saved from having a heart attack or stroke.
Other Considerations
Cost: Regular co-pay applies
Regimen: 1 pill once a day
Side effects: 9 out of 10 patients will have no side effects. 1 out of 10 patients may have nausea, diarrhea or constipation.
Muscle aching/stiffness: 5 out of 100 patients (some need to stop statins because of this)
Diabetes: Depending on the patients' individual risk factors and the dose prescribed, 1-2 patients out of 100 treated with statins will develop diabetes over ten years.
Muscle and kidney damage: 1 out of 20,000 patients (requires patients to stop statins)
Next
Document patient's choice and click continue
Statin Choice?
Yes
No
Undecided
CONTINUE

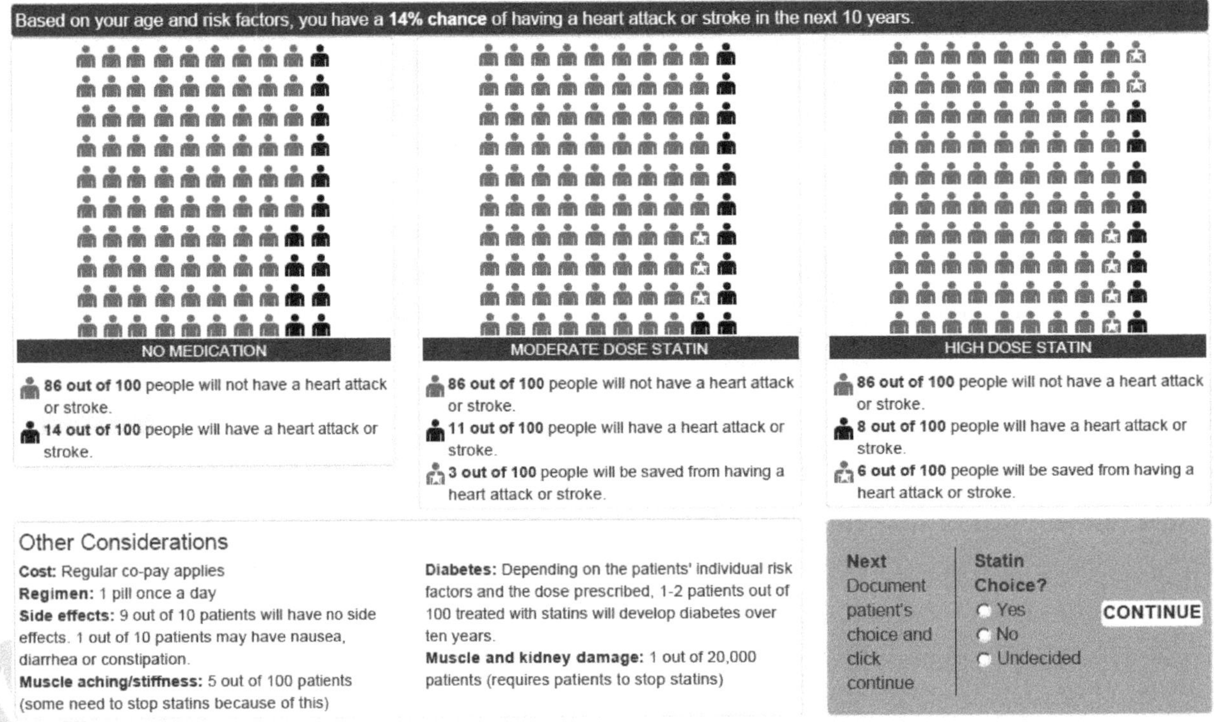

The graphic shows that, given a risk score of 14%, for every 100 people, during a 10-year period without taking statin drugs, 14 of the 100 will have a heart attack or stroke. This scenario is depicted in the panel on the left side of the graphic, labeled "no medication." The figures in light gray represent those who do not have a heart attack or stroke, whereas the dark gray figures represent the number of patients who do in fact suffer a heart attack or stroke. However, if all 100 people take a high-dose statin drug, as depicted in the panel on the right labeled "high-dose statin," only 8 of the 100 will have a heart attack or stroke; 8 ÷ 14 = 0.43; i.e., the "relative" risk reduction is a little over 40%.

That sounds like (and is) a lot, but the other way to look at risk is called "absolute" risk reduction. In this example, the original 10-year risk was 14%, and by taking the high-dose drug, we reduce an individual's risk to 8%; 14 - 8 = 6, for a 10-year absolute risk reduction of 6%. This is certainly a helpful thing, but is far less impressive sounding than the 40% relative risk reduction.

Usually, when we hear reports in the media or literature, people talk about relative risk reductions. However, as the example shows, what you really want to know before making a decision about taking a statin drug is the absolute risk reduction as it applies to your situation. In general, the higher your baseline risk, then the larger the absolute risk reduction, and the more likely you are to benefit from the medication.

Consider the following examples *(Bear in mind that taking the high-dose statin drug provides a relative risk reduction of 40%):* Imagine a patient who smokes, has high blood pressure and diabetes, as well as other cardiovascular risk factors. Suppose the patient has an overall 50% chance of heart attack or stroke during the next 10 years. Taking the high-dose statin drug would reduce that risk by 20 percentage points (absolute risk reduction) to 30%. That is a very substantial absolute risk reduction, and taking the medication would be worth it. On the other hand, if someone has only a 5% chance of heart attack or stroke during the next 10 years, taking the high-dose statin would reduce that risk by just 2 percentage points (absolute risk reduction) to 3%. That's not much of a gain, and taking the medication is probably not going to be worth it.

In other words, the decision as to whether or not to take the statin drug really depends on how high a risk you already have of heart attack or stroke. The higher your baseline risk, the greater your absolute risk reduction with taking the drug. The people at highest risk for heart attack are those who have already had one. Diabetic patients are also at very high risk. For this reason, we generally recommend the use of a statin medication to patients with heart disease and diabetes. For other patients, the decision to use a satin drug is an individual one, based upon the patient's overall cardiovascular risk, lifestyle, and individual preference.

If we do recommend a statin medication, we do so *in addition to,* not in place of, a good exercise regimen and a good diet. Studies have shown that, unfortunately, people taking statins tend to be sloppier with their diets.[128] The medical profession bears some responsibility, because not only some patients but also some physicians make the mistake of overemphasizing the use of medication at the expense of proper self-care. Diet, exercise, mind-body techniques, smoking cessation, and behavioral interventions for weight loss will all reduce the risk of cardiovascular disease. These should be emphasized first and should not take a backseat to pharmacotherapy.

The most commonly reported side effect from taking statin drugs is aches and pains in the muscles. A supplement called *coenzyme Q10* can help reduce this problem for some people who must take statin medications (see Chapter Eight).

CHAPTER FOURTEEN

IMPROVING CANCER CARE

How integrative medicine can help you take better care of yourself during cancer treatment.

We advise patients with cancer to work with their oncologists toward devising the most effective treatment plan for their particular circumstance. Modern cancer treatment protocols are often extremely effective and generally include some combination of surgery, chemotherapy, and radiation. These modalities, although often life-saving, unfortunately can have a lot of side effects. Complementary and integrative medicine can improve the care of patients with cancer by helping to both minimize the side effects of cancer treatment and improve quality of life. For example, we frequently recommend meditation training (see Chapter Seven) to patients undergoing cancer treatment. One study[129] done with breast cancer patients showed that when the practice of Transcendental Meditation was added to usual care, patients experienced improvements in overall quality of life, emotional well-being, and mental health. In addition to meditation, acupuncture helps to reduce nausea and vomiting for patients undergoing cancer chemotherapy.[130]

Diet plays an important role in both cancer prevention and in the management of side effects of cancer treatment. Researchers have found that consumption of a vegetarian diet is associated with both lower overall cancer rates[131] and reduced risk of colon cancer.[17] In addition, many patients with cancer suffer from poor appetite, and many have trouble maintaining their body weight. These problems can be caused either by the cancer condition itself or by the cancer treatments. A patient in this circumstance should focus on adhering to the guidelines for proper digestion detailed in earlier chapters (see Chapters Two to Four) and can benefit from favoring the dosha-specific diet pertinent to his/her constitutional type (see Chapter Five). In addition, many patients benefit from following a light diet. This is a diet consisting of nutritious foods that are readily digestible. A light diet can help patients keep up with their nutritional needs during times when eating and digesting food are difficult, such as when undergoing cancer therapies.

What is a light diet? The khichari recipe found in Chapter Three provides a great meal that is both nutritious and easy to digest. Cancer patients, especially those experiencing nausea, vomiting, or lack of appetite, should consider this a dietary staple. Other foods that can help in this context include boiled milk with ginger, stewed apples or pears, fresh vegetable juices, lassi, and soaked dates.

Another important source of nutrition for people with extremely low appetite and weak digestion is *kanji water*. This is essentially a rice water that you can drink when you are really having trouble keeping anything down.

KANJI WATER

Ingredients:

1 handful of basmati rice, rinsed
3 qt of water
1 tsp fresh grated ginger
½ tsp rock salt (from underground salt deposits rather than evaporated sea water)
Pinch of ground black pepper

Directions:

Boil the rice in the water for about an hour. Add spices and cook another 10 minutes. Remove from heat, strain, and drink the remaining fluid as tolerated.

Kanji water provides a good source of easily digested nutritional support when your appetite and digestion are extremely weak, such as during or immediately after cancer chemotherapy.

Foods to avoid when digestion is especially weak include cheese, eggs, and meats (if you prefer to include meat in your diet, a chicken broth or equivalent is okay). Avoid nut butters, raw vegetables, and cold drinks, including cold milk.

We often advise patients with cancer to take a traditional ayurvedic formulation called amrit kalash (available through MAPI www.mapi.com). The supplement consists of 2 separate preparations, an herbal paste, and an herbal tablet. The suggested dose is 1 teaspoon twice daily of the paste, and 1 tablet twice daily of the tablet. This is a traditional rasayana formula, and research has shown the supplements to have both anticancer[132,133] and antioxidant[134,135] properties. In addition, the supplements have been found to be effective in reducing liver toxicity associated with cancer chemotherapeutic drugs.[136] Note that some oncologists prefer that their patients not take antioxidants while undergoing cancer chemotherapy. This is because of theoretical concerns that an antioxidant supplement taken during cancer chemotherapy could render the chemotherapy program less effective. Although the matter is controversial, you should check with your oncologist first before deciding to take this or any other supplement while receiving cancer treatments.

Let's consider a few additional points regarding cancer prevention. If you smoke, you must quit. Smoking is associated not only with increased risk of lung cancer, but also with higher risk of many other types of cancer, including cancers of the head and neck, stomach, liver, pancreas, kidney, and cervix. We believe it best, to the extent practical, to limit pesticide exposure and to favor organic foods and produce (see Chapter Four). Although the data are controversial, pesticide exposure may be associated with the development of a range of cancers, including leukemia, lymphoma, and sarcoma.[137]

Complementary and integrative medicine can help improve cancer care. However, unproven alternative treatments are often a counterproductive distraction. Be wary of dramatic promises coupled with high price tags. Such unproven and unhelpful interventions burden the patient with needless additional expense, and, in the worst-case scenario, lure the patient from conventional treatments of proven benefit.

CHAPTER FIFTEEN

HORMONAL CHANGE

Healthy alternatives to pharmaceutical and hormonal therapies for women's health and menopause.

Patients present to our clinic with a range of women's health concerns. These include menstrual disorders (including premenstrual syndrome and painful or irregular menses), endometriosis, recurrent vaginal discharge, and menopausal symptoms.

We engage women between the ages of approximately 15 to 55 in an important discussion about *self-care during the menstrual period.* The time of the monthly menstrual period is a delicate and vulnerable period for the woman's physiology, during which proper self-care is essential. Although in modern society, many women have full-time jobs or busy careers and care for their family and home, we encourage them to focus as much as possible on rest and proper diet during menses. Doing so helps a woman avoid many of the most common gynecologic disorders and maintain optimal health.

We advise women to get as much rest as possible during the first 3 days of the menstrual period. Ideally, we would like to see each patient "check out and relax" during the first 3 days of menstrual flow. In a perfect world during these first 3 days the patient would not go into work, and would not be burdened with household duties. This of course is not feasible for most women in modern society, but even so, we encourage women to go as easy as possible, and to rest as much as is practical, during these first 3 days. This can mean canceling or rescheduling nonurgent appointments, as well as proactively avoiding unnecessary commitments. In addition, we advise women to observe a liquid fast for the first 1 to 2 days of the menstrual flow. The parameters for this are described in Chapter Eleven. Clear liquids, full liquids, and purees are all okay, but nothing solid by mouth for the first 1 to 2 days.

> **One of the first duties of the physician is to educate the masses not to take medicine.**
> — Sir William Osler

We encourage most women to avoid hormonal methods of birth control. For many patients, of course, the benefits of hormonal methods of birth control may outweigh the drawbacks. Even so, from the standpoint of maintaining physiologic balance, hormonal approaches to birth control interrupt the natural biorhythms of a woman's physiology. Bear in mind that according to ayurveda, the menstrual period serves as an important means of detoxification for the body. In other words, one function of menstruation is the elimination of ama, and any hormonal interventions that circumvent the menstrual flow altogether are especially worth avoiding when feasible. The use of condoms or barrier methods of birth control provide preferable contraceptive alternatives.

Additional lifestyle and dietary measures can help prevent and treat menstrual disorders. Women should favor specific spices in the diet including turmeric, cumin, hing, mustard seeds, and fenugreek seeds. Women should, likewise, to the extent possible eat a vegetarian diet (see Chapters Two through Five), including ample amounts of hot milk and ghee. Foods to avoid, especially during the menstrual flow, include leftover food, as well as heavy or hard-to-digest foods such as meat, fish, potato, butter, and cheese. We advise patients to avoid not only excess physical work, but also both travel and sexual intercourse during the menstrual period.

In Chapter Eleven, we reviewed potential ramifications of the blockage of apana vata (the component of vata dosha governing downward movement) in the context of our discussion of constipation. In the same way, if a woman on a habitual basis maintains too busy a schedule during the menstrual period, derangement of the natural downward flow of apana vata may result in an abnormal upward flow of energy. Health consequences include not only the development of endometriosis, menstrual irregularities, and other gynecologic disorders, but also headaches and other general or systemic symptoms. Maintaining rest and proper self-care during the menstrual period helps to maintain balance, prevent disease, and promote health.

A variety of supplements may be appropriate for women with menstrual-related problems and endometriosis; however, the correct prescription often requires physician consultation. A combination preparation called "smooth cycle" tablets, available from MAPI (www.mapi.com), has had good effect for many patients. Ashwagandha, 1 g to 2 g daily, can also be helpful.

For women with *recurrent vaginitis*, vaginal itching, or vaginal discharge, we recommend the behavioral regimen during the menstrual period as outlined above. In addition, the following 2 home remedies may be useful:

1. Triphala douche to be used 5 days after the end of the menstrual period. Purchase some triphala as a powder (see Chapter Eleven), or you can purchase triphala tablets and crush them. Boil 5 g of triphala in about 200 cc (6 to 8 ounces) of water, strain, and use as douche.
2. As an alternative (and especially if burning or dryness are predominant symptoms), apply 1 teaspoon of ghee (see Chapter Four) along with ½ teaspoon of raw honey to a tampon, insert intravaginally, keep overnight, then remove in the morning. (Note that it is important to apply more ghee than honey. Do not apply equal amounts of ghee and honey.)

Either of these remedies can be used as needed or periodically (every few weeks) for prevention.

Menopause represents the transition from the pitta to the vata season of life, and most menopausal symptoms can be attributed to vata imbalance. The prescribed program for balancing menopausal symptoms thus focuses on balancing vata dosha, using the range of modalities including diet (see Chapters Two to Five), daily routine (see Chapter Six), and mind body approaches (see Chapter Seven). We generally advise a light vata-balancing diet (see Chapter Five), although a pitta diet may be indicated in the setting of prominent hot flashes. Women should favor a diet rich in whole grains that provide phytoestrogen support. These include amaranth, bulgur wheat, rice, barley, quinoa, and rye. To promote the balance of vata dosha, maintenance of a regular routine, including regular exercise, is key. To relieve hot flashes the patient can perform the daily oil massage (see Chapter Twelve) with coconut oil, which is more cooling, as opposed to sesame oil, which is more heating. Including in the diet some stewed apples or pears at breakfast time also helps to relieve and prevent hot flashes.

Hormone replacement therapy (HRT) refers to the use of female hormones like estrogen and progesterone to help ward off symptoms of menopause. Taking these hormones can have side effects and should be avoided for most patients. Side effects of HRT include increased risk of heart attack, stroke, blood clots, and breast cancer. Many women turn to "bioidentical hormone" therapy as an alternative to prescription hormones, but we likewise advise most patients against the use of this approach. Bioidentical hormone replacement technically refers to the idea of using a hormone that is structurally identical to a hormone produced normally by the body. People also use the term to refer to the ingestion or topical application of individually compounded combinations of multiple hormones, including estrogens, progesterone, testosterone, and others. However, the body does not naturally produce substantial amounts of these hormones at the menopausal stage of life, nor is it natural to boost menopausal women's levels with hormonal creams, tablets, patches, implants, or pills. Bioidentical hormone therapy holds the same risks as any other approach to hormone replacement. In addition, there is less regulatory oversight of the quality and potency of compounded bioidentical hormone preparations.[138] We usually advise avoidance of hormonal replacement therapy of any type for perimenopausal and postmenopausal women.

A number of herbal supplements may be helpful for women as they approach menopause. We target such recommendations to the specific menopausal symptoms reported by the patient. For example, many women report anxiety or depression associated with menopause, which we address using the protocols reviewed in Chapter Twelve. In addition, some herbal approaches may be helpful for alleviating menopausal hot flashes. "Hot flash relief" tablets, available from MAPI (www.mapi.com), contain shatavari and other ayurvedic herbal ingredients that have been effective for many of our patients. Black cohosh is an herbal supplement that has been shown to be effective for managing menopausal hot flashes in several clinical trials.[139] The supplement has been safely used in studies lasting up to one year. Dosage will vary depending on the preparation or product.

You can also make a homemade herbal decoction that can help with menopausal hot flashes. Add ¼ teaspoon of cumin seeds, ¼ teaspoon of coriander seeds, ¼ teaspoon of fennels seeds, ½ teaspoon of food-grade rose petals, and 2 to 4 cups of hot water, to a thermos and sip warm throughout the day.

Sometimes, despite appropriate diet, herbs, and behavioral and mind-body approaches, menopausal symptoms persist. In such cases we can sometimes trace the cause to ama accumulation, and the patient may benefit from ama pachana procedures (see Chapter Twelve).

Prevention of osteoporosis is a main priority for women in the postmenopausal phase of life. When osteoporosis sets in, the bones grow more brittle, placing the patient at increased risk of fractures of the hip and back. What can be done to preserve bone health? Exercising on a regular basis helps preserve bone strength. If you smoke, you must quit. Additionally, physicians advise both vitamin D supplementation and calcium supplementation. We recommend vitamin D in doses of 1000 IU to 2000 IU daily, and calcium in doses of 1000 mg to 1500 mg daily. We also recommend that patients take measures to reduce the risk of falling. For example, studies have shown that Tai Chi training (see Chapter Seven) helps reduce the risk of falls.[140]

Physicians commonly recommend alendronate (Fosamax) as a medication that effectively reduces the risk of bone fractures in women with osteoporosis. Patients take the medication once weekly first thing in the morning on an empty stomach. During a period of 3 to 4 years, alendronate offers relative risk reductions (see Chapter Thirteen) for vertebral fractures in the range of 40% to 50%, but absolute risk reductions only in the range of 2% to 8%.[141] The main side effect of alendronate is upper gastrointestinal irritation including acid reflux. Osteonecrosis (bone breakdown) of the jaw is another potential problem that can also occur as a side effect of alendronate, but this is rare.

Strontium is an element that people take orally for treatment of osteoporosis. Researchers have shown one preparation, strontium ranelate, to be effective at reducing the frequency of bone fractures.[142] Strontium ranelate is available as a prescription medication in many countries but is not available in the US. Another strontium preparation, strontium citrate, is available in supplements in the US but its efficacy has not been proven.

Many patients present to our clinic with concerns about *hormonal balance*. Some of these patients have symptoms that can in fact be attributed to low or high levels of thyroid, adrenal, or other hormones. Most of the time, the process of diagnosing, or ruling out, such endocrine conditions is straightforward and can be accomplished by obtaining a history and physical examination, along with a few tests. More commonly, the patient's focus on hormonal function is misplaced. When a patient's symptoms persist in the face of normal hormonal testing, we advise not a hormonal supplement but rather a change in perspective. Shifting the attention in the direction of diet, exercise, stress reduction, improving digestion, and balancing the doshas provides the patient with fresh insight and direction.

Healthy aging is a priority concern not only for postmenopausal women, but for men as well. The last part of life (from around age 60 and older) is the vata season of life, and health disorders related to aging mostly represent imbalances of vata dosha. We advise mind/body practice (see Chapter Seven), a vata-balancing diet (see Chapter Five), and a regular routine (see Chapter Six) to all patients. In addition, we strongly encourage both a regular program of physical exercise as well as a focus on keeping one's mind active and sharp. Reading, volunteering, completing crossword puzzles, taking a university course, and learning a foreign language all contribute to maintaining mental acuity. To help improve or maintain mental function, we often recommend *Brahmi (Bacopa),* an ayurvedic herb traditionally used for this indication (see Chapter Eight). *Gingko biloba* is a supplement that some people recommend to prevent or treat dementia. Although the data remain controversial, overall it seems that Ginkgo may help improve cognitive symptoms for some patients with dementia.[143] A typical dose is 120 mg to 240 mg daily of the standardized extract.

PATIENT TESTIMONIAL

"The nearby grocery store had been renovated to accommodate a glorious organic produce section. One of the familiar check-out clerks was on duty and surprised me by saying, 'You buy healthier food than anyone else, and I see hundreds and hundreds of customers. You look extremely healthy and energetic. Please tell me what you eat.' I told her a little. A few days later, as she was going on break, she rushed up and with interest, and sincerely asked me to expand. Dr. Elder had said that what he suggested I eat could be generic, so I seriously and forcefully told her exactly what Dr. Elder had told me to eat and not to eat. We talked until she understood, probably past her break time.

A few weeks later, from 20 feet away I received a never-to-be-forgotten impression. She had lost weight and was well proportioned. Her skin was simply glowing, luminous, and radiant. She said she had been doing 100% of what Dr. Elder prescribed and her favorite part was eating rolled oats boiled in 2% milk for dinner every night. She was now passionate about the diet and her health. It showed and she glowed.

Once utterly terrified of the kitchen, I am now able to prepare nutritious whole food meals, fulfilling and satisfying. This is so much the case that cravings have fallen away, as has any desire to eat anything other than what Dr. Elder said. Breakfast, lunch, and dinner are prepped and cooked day after day, month after month, with remarkable enthusiasm and increased refinement. 'It just flows,' as Dr. Elder said.

Chronic indigestion has been replaced by near perfect digestion. Allied ayurvedic disciplines are fun and profound. 'The body of one who uses oil massage regularly does not become affected much, even if subjected to accidental injuries or strenuous work. By using oil massage daily, a person becomes strong, charming, and least affected by old age.' — Charaka Samhita

My energy level is continuously high, so much so that recently someone said, 'You wow 'em at the gym.' Regularly people think I am 20 to 25 years younger than my actual 75 years, and I can honestly say old age has not yet risen on the horizon."

CHAPTER SIXTEEN

LOSE YOUR TV

Topics related to the care of children, including ADHD, vaccinations, and respiratory congestion.

Attention Deficit Hyperactivity Disorder: ADHD

Although some children with ADHD will require medication, we maintain that contemporary medical practice overemphasizes pharmacotherapy, and most children should be approached using behavioral and holistic approaches. Following are some suggestions and guidelines:

The mind-body approaches reviewed in Chapter Seven, as well as the herbal and behavior remedies presented at the end of Chapter Twelve (section on anxiety), are applicable to and often effective for ADHD. We generally halve the dosage of the supplements for children under 12.

ADHD often reflects problems with the amount or type of attention the child is receiving. When a child shows symptoms of ADHD, we encourage the family to review and to consider some potentially sensitive lifestyle issues. Is the child overscheduled? Are both parents working? What steps can be taken to increase "down time" for the child? What practical options can be devised to provide the child with more individual attention from parents, grandparents, or other family members?

Excessive electronic media exposure can aggravate attention problems. Studies show an association between electronic media use and increased attention problems in childhood.[144] Unfortunately, the matter no longer involves just television. The seemingly uncontrolled proliferation of computers, smart phones, and video game consoles introduces additional complexity and urgency to this issue. The American Academy of Pediatrics recommends limitations on digital media use for children age 2 to 5 years to no more than 1 hour per day.[145] Electronic media exposure for children younger than 2 years old should be avoided altogether.

The Academy suggests a variety of steps that can be taken to help limit the media exposure of children. These include:

- Families can develop a media-use plan with specific guidelines and goals for each child and parent.
- Physicians should educate parents about brain development in the early years and the importance of hands-on and unstructured activities for developing social and emotional skills.
- When children are using media, parents should use the app, or watch the movie, or play the game along with the child. This is how children learn best. Avoid letting children use media by themselves.
- Avoid programming that is too fast paced or violent.
- Turn off television and media when not in use.
- Allow no screens or devices in the bedroom. Stop using screens at least an hour before bed.
- As a general principle, avoid using media as a babysitter, or as a systemic strategy for calming your child.
- Keep meal times screen and media free.

In addition to the association with attention problems, media use in early childhood has also been linked to cognitive, language, and social and emotional delays.[146] Other health problems associated with media exposure in young children include obesity and sleep problems. The bottom line on media use for young children is, "less is more."

VACCINES

The issue of v*accinations* stirs up plenty of controversy and emotion. People have misidentified the central issue, which has less to do with science than with restoring dialogue and trust. We reassure our patients that vaccination represents an important strategy for preserving both individual and public health, and that vaccines generally are both effective and safe. Diseases such as polio and tetanus are real, and are now entirely preventable, through vaccination.

However, many patients remain justifiably skeptical about a dogmatic, one-size-fits-all approach to vaccinating. The vaccination schedule circulated by public health authorities provides an important guideline, but many patients remain suspicious that some of the shots may be unnecessary, and not without reason. In the US, the required number of vaccine doses for children in the first two years of life (49) is the highest of all the G8 countries and is more than 50% higher than the required number of doses in France.[147] As another example, the current recommendation by the Advisory Committee on Immunization Practices (ACIP) in the US is to administer two separate pneumonia vaccines, both PPSV23 and the newer PCV13, to all adults age 65 years or older. This approach has thus been aggressively implemented in many clinics. However, "the recommendation to give both PPSV23 and PCV13 to high-risk adults is far more costly than recommending PPSV23 alone. In addition, adherence to a two-vaccine regimen is likely to be poorer than adherence to a one-vaccine regimen. Despite the strength of the current ACIP recommendation, data supporting this approach are meager."[148] Finally, recall that during the 1990s, the prevalent view in biomedicine was that every woman older than age 50 years needed hormone replacement therapy. We later learned that the health risks of hormone replacement therapy may outweigh the benefits (see Chapter Fifteen), and the medical profession dramatically reversed its position. Against such a backdrop, public skepticism is inevitable. Current vaccine recommendations need not be viewed as divine revelation etched in stone. A more nuanced, patient-centered approach is required, emphasizing dialogue, education, and shared decision making.

RESPIRATORY ISSUES

Tips For Reducing Respiratory Congestion

Childhood represents the kapha season of life, and children are thus prone to imbalances of kapha dosha. Kapha imbalance, in turn, commonly presents as excessive mucus production in the form of allergies, ear infections, upper respiratory infections, asthma, otitis media, and the like. The following guidelines can help reduce or prevent these symptoms, and are applicable not only to children, but also to adults.

Avoid kapha-aggravating foods and beverages. Specifically, radically limit intake of foods and beverages that are cold and/or sweet. In other words, if you have a sinus infection, don't eat ice cream! If your child or grandchild has nasal congestion or frequent middle ear infections, do not give him or her cold juice or cold milk out of the refrigerator. Such beverages will increase kapha, cause more congestion, and may aggravate or even represent the cause of the child's symptoms.

As a general principle, avoid sugar-sweetened beverages altogether. No soft drinks and no juice drinks, period. Fresh fruit is great, but avoid store-bought fruit juices, especially when cold. You can have fresh-squeezed juices at home in limited amounts, but as always consume these at room temperature, not cold.

Reduce or avoid puffy breads. Instead, favor flatbreads such as pita bread, chapatis, or tortillas. In any case, you should always try to toast breads before eating.

Follow a kapha-balancing diet, as described in Chapter Five.

At the first sign of upper respiratory symptoms, prepare the following home remedy:

Mix together a few tablespoons of raw honey with a few teaspoons of turmeric. Stir to make a honey and turmeric paste. Take 1 teaspoon of the honey-turmeric paste 2 to 4 times a day.

Try the "spicy milk" recipe described in Chapter Four.

Drink the following homemade decoction: Place in a thermos: ¼ teaspoon cumin seeds, ¼ teaspoon coriander seeds, ¼ teaspoon fennel seeds, a pinch of black pepper, and a little salt to taste. Add 2 to 4 cups of boiling hot water, then sip throughout the day.

Gargle with hot water, salt, and turmeric.

Inhale moist steam with eucalyptus oil.

Finally, we should reemphasize that as children are prone to respiratory congestion, parents should avoid giving their children kapha-aggravating foods and beverages. The common practice of serving kids lots of cold milk and cold juice represents an underrecognized cause of pediatric health problems. Before giving your children a glass of milk, remember to boil the milk first, ideally with a pinch of turmeric or a slice of ginger, then serve it hot. No cold milk for kids. No cold juice. And *especially* no sugar-sweetened beverages!

CHAPTER SEVENTEEN

CONCLUSION

The Picture of Health

About 20 years ago, I attended a weekend ayurvedic clinical update for physicians in the San Francisco Bay area. For many years I had been a heavy coffee drinker, relying on generous portions of caffeine to get me through the long clinic days and the difficult overnight hospital call shifts. I, of course, knew that the coffee wasn't good for me, especially in the face of my strong pitta constitution. Although I liked the quick pick-up, excess coffee typically left me prone to irritability, temper flares, and acid indigestion. Even so, I held drinking plenty of good coffee while seeing patients as a cherished habit, dating back to medical school.

On the other hand, drinking coffee at the ayurvedic seminar would be viewed as highly unfashionable. Caffeinated drinks are off the menu. Not surprisingly, however, I wasn't the only physician in attendance suffering from a caffeine obsession. As most of us know, discontinuing coffee can be an uncomfortable experience. Specifically, caffeine withdrawal can cause a nasty headache. Mercifully, the course organizers wanted to help participants avoid feeling uncomfortable during the meeting. At the back of the room, by the hot water thermos, they placed not only the usual assortment of herbal teas, but also a jar of instant coffee. That way, balance of the doshas notwithstanding, we caffeine addicts could get our fix and enjoy the course.

Rather than publicly embarrassing myself by openly drinking instant coffee at an ayurvedic training seminar, I elected to stick with the herbal teas come what may. The course materials taught us about self-care and natural medicine, and I found the seminar both informative and inspiring. Of course, I had an awful headache the entire weekend. After this course, however, I was finally ready to quit. I had lost my appetite for the drug. Since that weekend, as far as caffeinated beverages go, I have hardly had a sip. After consuming all that coffee for all those years, attending this course brought me to a place where I simply no longer wanted to use the drug. I could feel and see that the cons outweighed the pros. The bad habit just fell away.

Different people adopt various approaches to behavior change. What is the best approach to breaking a bad habit, such as cigarette smoking? Some like to drop a bad habit "cold turkey," whereas others prefer a slow steady taper. What about the introduction of good habits? One approach to eliminating bad habits is to adopt good ones! Often times, by adopting the proper health-promoting routine and diet, bad habits will naturally evaporate. Just as plowing and fertilizing a field optimizes growth of the crop, so do proper diet, routine, exercise, and health practices set the stage for ideal healthy functioning of the mind and body. As the physiology grows more refined, the negative side effects of, say, a nicotine or alcohol addiction grow more acutely obvious, until the continuation of the habit becomes untenable. The physiology has grown too sensitive to the side effects of the drug.

We have presented a lot of ideas in this book but the patient should not feel overwhelmed. When someone is ready to take steps to improve his or her health, what should be done first? We encourage patients to go one step at a time. Select an idea or lifestyle change that appeals to you, and makes sense to you, and try it. For example, start having your main meal at midday, and reducing the food at night. Try this for just 2 weeks. Probably, you will notice a big improvement in how you feel. Then the choice is yours. Do you want to continue the new routine and feel better, or is it worth it to eat a lot at night, and feel worse?

The normal state for all of us is to be healthy and to thrive. Illness represents a mistake. What lifestyle markers indicate both the cause and effect of ideal health? What does that picture look like? Ayurveda, the "science of lifespan," provides answers. We simply implement the plan, and over time, good health will naturally set in, and bad habits and disease will evaporate.

The template is straightforward. Wake up early every morning, ideally by 6 a.m. Get some exercise, like a brisk walk, or whatever you enjoy, first thing each morning. Have a good nutritious lunch every day as your main meal. Get to bed early, ideally by 10 p.m. The next day, repeat, and so on. Early to bed, early to rise, get some exercise in the morning, and have a decent lunch! That's really all there is to it. The picture of health! This simple routine sets your body in sync with nature, establishing the foundation for the normal functioning of the physiology, which is ideal health.

You can, and should, additionally add the simple, powerful self-help modalities described in earlier chapters, when it seems natural for you to do so. You can introduce a mind-body practice (see Chapter Seven), ideally in the morning and evening every day. A daily abhyanga oil massage with sesame oil (see Chapter Twelve) can be done before your shower every morning. Adopting these practices will accelerate and maintain ideal balance. Once you are in the good habit, you won't want to stop.

Wake up by 6 a.m., meditate, exercise, then do the oil massage and take a shower. Have a good nutritious lunch. Meditate again in the late afternoon. Get to bed by 10 p.m. The next day, repeat, and so on. There you have it, the picture of health! With this routine in place, health and vitality will come naturally.

Eat and drink foods and beverages that support, rather than impede, your progress. A balanced diet, emphasizing whole grains, legumes, cooked vegetables, fresh fruit, and the judicious use of dairy products provides for a delicious cuisine that is wholesome, health promoting, and nutritionally complete. You can use as a guide whichever dosha-specific diet is appropriate for your body type or specific health challenge. These diets allow you to select the specific spices and foods that will most effectively restore and maintain optimum balance and health.

Herbal supplements can be added to accelerate progress. The formulations serve to improve digestion, eliminate ama, balance the doshas, and promote the body's innate healing mechanisms without toxic side effects. Other practitioner-administered modalities should be layered on top when needed. Detoxification procedures, acupuncture, and spinal or soft tissue manipulation can all play a vital role in treating illness and restoring health.

When disease has set in, medications or surgery often provide the most sensible and powerful solutions. Even so, a good routine and dynamic self-care regimen will enhance the effectiveness of conventional medicine interventions, maximizing the patient's ability to withstand any side effects of treatment. The self-care sets the stage for the patient to best benefit from the medication, or to most quickly recover from the surgery.

So what is the daily routine, what are the exercise patterns, and how does one use diet, mind-body techniques, and herbal supplements in ways that most effectively support health and longevity over the long haul? Now you know! All that remains is for you to do it, one step at a time. Ideal health will inevitably manifest.

Get the picture!

RESOURCES

Health tips and information about ayurveda

If you like this book and want to keep learning, check out our website and blog at: www.PictureofHealthMDs.com

Ayurvedic herbs and supplements

We generally direct our patients to one of several good herbal suppliers when purchasing ayurvedic supplements. Reliable online distributors include:

Maharishi Ayurveda Products International (MAPI)
www.mapi.com or 1-800-ALL-VEDA
MAPI holds both GMP (Good Manufacturing Practices) and IS0-9001 quality certifications. In addition, many of the products are USDA-certified organic.

Banyan Botanicals
www.banyanbotanicals.com or 1-800-953-6424
Nearly all of the bulk herbs sold through this site are USDA-certified organically grown.

Ayurvedic training

Information about high-quality distance learning training modules in ayurveda for health care professionals can be found at:

Institute of Ayurveda Medical Education
www.ayurveda-courses.org

Pancha karma

A number of reputable centers in North America provide pancha karma treatments, including:

The Raj
1734 Jasmine Ave
Fairfield, Iowa 52556
641-472-9580
www.theraj.com

The Ayurvedic Institute
11311 Menaul Blvd NE
Albuquerque, New Mexico 87122
505-291-9698
www.ayurveda.com/panchakarma/overview

GLOSSARY

Ama: Digestive toxins. The byproduct of incomplete or improper digestion.

Ayurveda: The traditional health care system of India, widely viewed as perhaps the oldest continuously practiced system of holistic medicine in the world.

Alternative medicine: The use of nonmainstream health care approaches as a replacement for, or instead of, conventional medicine. (In general we avoid this term in the book, just as we avoid using this approach in our practice.)

Complementary medicine: The use of nonmainstream health care approaches together with, or as a supplement to, conventional medicine.

Conventional medicine: Today's mainstream approach to health care (also known as "Allopathic" medicine).

Dosha: Psychometabolic principle, or humor. According to ayurveda, health is a state of balance and disease is a state of imbalance of the three doshas.

Holistic: An approach to health care that considers the whole person, taking into account not only physical symptoms, but also mental, social, and spiritual dimensions.

Integrative medicine: Bringing conventional and complementary medicine approaches together in a coordinated way.

Kapha: The dosha governing all structure and lubrication.

Ojas: The product of healthy digestion: sweet, light, and nutritious, and nourishing to all the tissues of the body.

Pitta: The dosha governing heat, digestion, and metabolism.

Prakriti: An individual's ayurvedic body type.

Vata: The dosha governing movement.

Vikriti: The current state of imbalance of the doshas for an individual patient.

BIBLIOGRAPHY

1. Dillbeck MC. The effect of the transcendental meditation technique on anxiety level. J Clin Psychol 1977 Oct;33(4):1076-8. DOI: https://doi.org/10.1002/1097-4679(197710)33:4<1076::aid-jclp2270330435>3.0.co;2-b.
2. Sharma HM, Dwivedi C, Satter BC, Abou-Issa H. Antineoplastic properties of Maharishi Amrit Kalash [MAK-7], an ayurvedic food supplement, against 7,12-dimethylbenz (a) anthracene-induced mammary tumors in rats. J Res Educ Indian Med 1991;10(3):1-8.
3. Sharma HM, Hanna AN, Kauffman EM, Newman HA. Inhibition of human low-density lipoprotein oxidation in vitro by Maharishi Ayur-Veda herbal mixtures. Pharmacol Biochem Behav 1992 Dec;43(4):1175-82. DOI: https://doi.org/10.1016/0091-3057(92)90500-f.
4. Sharma PV, translator. Caraka Samhita. Varanasi, India: Chaukhambha Orientalia; 1981.
5. Sharma H, Chandola HM, Singh G, Basisht G. Utilization of Ayurveda in health care: An approach for prevention, health promotion, and treatment of disease. Part 1—Ayurveda, the science of life. J Altern Complement Med 2007 Nov;13(9):1011-9. DOI: https://doi.org/10.1089/acm.2007.7017-A.
6. Sharma H, Chandola HM, Singh G, Basisht G. Utilization of Ayurveda in health care: An approach for prevention, health promotion, and treatment of disease. Part 2—Ayurveda in primary health care. J Altern Complement Med 2007 Dec;13(10):1135-50. DOI: https://doi.org/10.1089/acm.2007.7017-B.
7. Elder C, Aickin M, Bauer V, Cairns J, Vuckovic N. Randomized trial of a whole-system ayurvedic protocol for type 2 diabetes. Altern Ther Health Med 2006 Sep-Oct;12(5):24-30.
8. Dunlap C, Hanes D, Elder C, Nygaard C, Zwicky H. Reliability of self-reported constitutional questionnaires in ayurveda diagnosis. J Ayurveda Integr Med 2017 Oct-Dec;8(4):257-62. DOI: https://doi.org/10.1016/j.jaim.2017.04.011.
9. Farhadi A, Banan A, Fields J, Keshavarzian A. Intestinal barrier: An interface between health and disease. J Gastroenterol Hepatol 2003 May;18(5):479-97. DOI: https://doi.org/10.1046/j.1440-1746.2003.03032.x.
10. Kuehn BM. Resetting the circadian clock might boost metabolic health. JAMA 2017 Apr 4;317(13):1303-5. DOI: https://doi.org/10.1001/jama.2017.0653.
11. Sone Y, Hyun KJ, Nishimura S, Lee YA, Tokura H. Effects of dim or bright-light exposure during the daytime on human gastrointestinal activity. Chronobiol Int 2003 Jan;20(1):123-33. DOI: https://doi.org/10.1081/cbi-120017688.
12. Stenvers DJ, Jonkers CF, Fliers E, Bisschop PH, Kalsbeek A. Nutrition and the circadian timing system. Prog Brain Res 2012;199:359-76. DOI: https://doi.org/10.1016/B978-0-444-59427-3.00020-4.
13. Cagampang FR, Bruce KD. The role of the circadian clock system in nutrition and metabolism. Br J Nutr 2012 Aug;108(3):381-92. DOI: https://doi.org/10.1017/S0007114512002139.
14. St-Onge M, Ard J, Baskin ML, et al; American Heart Association Obesity Committee of the Council on Lifestyle and Cardiometabolic Health; Council on Cardiovascular Disease in the Young; Council on Clinical Cardiology; and Stroke Council. Meal timing and frequency: Implications for cardiovascular disease prevention: A scientific statement from the American Heart Association. Circulation 2017 Feb 28;135(9):e96-e121. DOI: https://doi.org/10.1161/CIR.0000000000000476.
15. Sharma H, Clark C. Contemporary ayurveda: Medicine and research in maharishi ayurveda. Philadelphia, PA: Churchill Livingstone; 1998.
16. Orlich MJ, Singh PN, Sabaté J, et al. Vegetarian dietary patterns and mortality in Adventist Health Study 2. JAMA Intern Med 2013 Jul 8;173(13):1230-8. DOI: https://doi.org/10.1001/jamainternmed.2013.6473.
17. Orlich MJ, Singh PN, Sabaté J, et al. Vegetarian dietary patterns and the risk of colorectal cancers. JAMA Intern Med 2015 May;175(5):767-76. DOI: https://doi.org/10.1001/jamainternmed.2015.59.
18. Tommasini A, Not T, Kiren V, et al. Mass screening for coeliac disease using antihuman transglutaminase antibody assay. Arch Dis Child 2004 Jun;89(6):512-5. DOI: https://doi.org/10.1136/adc.2003.029603.

19. Molina-Infante J, Santolaria S, Sanders DS, Fernández-Bañares F. Systematic review: Noncoeliac gluten sensitivity. Aliment Pharmacol Ther 2015 May;41(9):807-20. DOI: https://doi.org/10.1111/apt.13155.
20. Gibson PR, Shepherd SJ. Food choice as a key management strategy for functional gastrointestinal symptoms. Am J Gastroenterol 2012 May;107(5):657-66. DOI: https://doi.org/10.1038/ajg.2012.49.
21. Skodje GI, Sarna VK, Minelle IH, et al. Fructan, rather than gluten, induces symptoms in patients with self-reported non-celiac gluten sensitivity. Gastroenterology 2018 Feb;154(3):529-539.e2. DOI: https://doi.org/10.1053/j.gastro.2017.10.040.
22. Scrimshaw NS, Murray EB. The acceptability of milk and milk products in populations with a high prevalence of lactose intolerance. Am J Clin Nutr 1988 Oct;48(4 Suppl):1083-159. DOI: https://doi.org/10.1093/ajcn/48.4.1142.
23. Bu G, Luo Y, Chen F, Liu K, Zhu T. Milk processing as a tool to reduce cow's milk allergenicity: A mini-review. Dairy Sci Technol 2013 May;93(3):211-23.DOI: https://doi.org/10.1007/s13594-013-0113-x.
24. Kim JS, Nowak-Węgrzyn A, Sicherer SH, Noone S, Moshier EL, Sampson HA. Dietary baked milk accelerates the resolution of cow's milk allergy in children. J Allergy Clin Immunol 2011 Jul;128(1):125-131.e2. DOI: https://doi.org/10.1016/j.jaci.2011.04.036.
25. Young VB. The role of the microbiome in human health and disease: An introduction for clinicians. BMJ 2017 Mar 15;356:j831. DOI: https://doi.org/10.1136/bmj.j831.
26. Weaver CM. Should dairy be recommended as part of a healthy vegetarian diet? Point. Am J Clin Nutr 2009 May;89(5):1634S-7S. DOI: https://doi.org/10.3945/ajcn.2009.267360.
27. Craig WJ. Health effects of vegan diets. Am J Clin Nutr 2009 May;89(5):1627S-33S. DOI: https://doi.org/10.3945/ajcn.2009.26736N.
28. van Vreeswijk H, Pameyer JH. Inducing cataract in post-mortem pig eyes for cataract surgery training purposes. J Cataract Refract Surg 1998 Jan;24(1):17-8. DOI: https://doi.org/10.1016/s0886-3350(98)80068-0.
29. Quan R, Yang C, Rubinstein S, et al. Effects of microwave radiation on anti-infective factors in human milk. Pediatrics 1992 Apr;89(4 Pt 1):667-9.
30. George DF, Bilek MM, McKenzie DR. Non-thermal effects in the microwave induced unfolding of proteins observed by chaperone binding. Bioelectromagnetics 2008 May;29(4):324-30. DOI: https://doi.org/10.1002/bem.20382.
31. Vallejo F, Tomás-Barberán FA, García-Viguera C. Phenolic compound contents in edible parts of broccoli inflorescences after domestic cooking. Journal of the Science of Food and Agriculutre 2003 Oct;83(14):1511-6. DOI: https://doi.org/10.1002/jsfa.1585.
32. Yuan G, Sun B, Yuan J, Wang CM. Effects of different cooking methods on health-promoting compounds of broccoli. J Zhejiang Univ Sci B 2009 Aug;10(8):580-8. DOI: https://doi.org/10.1631/jzus.B0920051.
33. EWG. Dirty dozen: EWG's 2018 shopper's guide to pesticides in produce [Internet]. Washington, DC: Enviromental Work Group; 2018 [accessed 2018 Jul 21]. Available from: www.ewg.org/foodnews/dirty_dozen_list.php.
34. Annapoorani A, Anilakumar K, Khanum F, Murthy NA, Bawa AS. Studies on the physicochemical characteristics of heated honey, honey mixed with ghee and their food consumption pattern by rats. Ayu 2010 Apr-Jun;31(2):141-6. DOI: https://doi.org/ 10.4103/0974-8520.72363.
35. Toxnet. 5-Hydroxymethyl-2-furfuraldehyde [Internet]. Washington, DC: National Library of Medicine; 2011 Aug 29 [updated 2012 Apr 26; cited 2017 May 3]. Available from: https://toxnet.nlm.nih.gov/cgi-bin/sis/search/a?dbs+hsdb:@term+@DOCNO+7982.
36. Lampe JW. Spicing up a vegetarian diet: Chemopreventive effects of phytochemicals. Am J Clin Nutr 2003 Sep;78(3 Suppl):579S-83S. DOI: https://doi.org/10.1093/ajcn/78.3.579S.
37. Van Proeyen K, Szlufcik K, Nielens H, et al. Training in the fasted state improves glucose tolerance during fat-rich diet. J Physiol 2010 Nov 1;588(Pt 21):4289-302. DOI: https://doi.org/10.1113/jphysiol.2010.196493.
38. Kecklund G, Axelsson J. Health consequences of shift work and insufficient sleep. BMJ 2016 Nov 1;355:i5210. DOI: https://doi.org/10.1136/bmj.i5210.
39. Lin X, Chen W, Wei F, Ying M, Wei W, Xie X. Night-shift work increases morbidity of breast cancer and all-cause mortality: A meta-analysis of 16 prospective cohort studies. Sleep Med 2015 Nov;16(11):1381-7. DOI: https://doi.org/10.1016/j.sleep.2015.02.543.

40. Wallace RK. Physiological effects of transcendental meditation. Science 1970 Mar 27;167(3926):1751-4. DOI: https://doi.org/10.1126/science.167.3926.1751.
41. Elder C. Meditation. Perm J 2005 Summer;9(3):67-8.
42. Travis F, Shear J. Focused attention, open monitoring and automatic self-transcending: Categories to organize meditations from Vedic, Buddhist and Chinese traditions. Conscious Cogn 2010 Dec;19(4):1110-8. DOI: https://doi.org/10.1016/j.concog.2010.01.007.
43. Brook RD, Appel LJ, Rubenfire M, et al; American Heart Association Professional Education Committee of the Council for High Blood Pressure Research, Council on Cardiovascular and Stroke Nursing, Council on Epidemiology and Prevention, and Council on Nutrition, Physical Activity. Beyond medications and diet: Alternative approaches to lowering blood pressure: A scientific statement from the American Heart Association. Hypertension 2013 Jun;61(6):1360-83. DOI: https://doi.org/ 10.1161/HYP.0b013e318293645f.
44. Nidich SI, Rainforth MV, Haaga DA, et al. A randomized controlled trial on effects of the Transcendental Meditation program on blood pressure, psychological distress, and coping in young adults. Am J Hypertens 2009 Dec;22(12):1326-31. DOI: https://doi.org/10.1038/ajh.2009.184.
45. Orme-Johnson DW, Barnes VA. Effects of the transcendental meditation technique on trait anxiety: A meta-analysis of randomized controlled trials. J Altern Complement Med 2014 May;20(5):330-41. DOI: https://doi.org/10.1089/acm.2013.0204.
46. Elder C, Nidich S, Moriarty F, Nidich R. Effect of transcendental meditation on employee stress, depression, and burnout: A randomized controlled study. Perm J 2014 Winter;18(1):19-23. DOI: https://doi.org/10.7812/TPP/13-102.
47. Chou R, Deyo R, Friedly J, et al. Nonpharmacologic therapies for low back pain: A systematic review for an American College of Physicians Clinical Practice Guideline. Ann Intern Med 2017 Apr 4;166(7):493-505. DOI: https://doi.org/ 10.7326/M16-2459.
48. Zhang MF, Wen YS, Liu WY, Peng LF, Wu XD, Liu QW. Effectiveness of mindfulness-based therapy for reducing anxiety and depression in patients with cancer: A meta-analysis. Medicine (Baltimore) 2015 Nov;94(45):e0897-0. DOI: https://doi.org/10.1097/md.0000000000000897.
49. Cheung C, Park J, Wyman JF. Effects of yoga on symptoms, physical function, and psychosocial outcomes in adults with osteoarthritis: A focused review. Am J Phys Med Rehabil 2016 Feb;95(2):139-51. DOI: https://doi.org/10.1097/PHM.0000000000000408.
50. Kligler B, Teets R, Quick M. Complementary/integrative therapies that work: A review of the evidence. Am Fam Physician 2016 Sep 1;94(5):369-74.
51. Wang C, Schmid CH, Iversen MD, et al. Comparative effectiveness of tai chi versus physical therapy for knee osteoarthritis: A randomized trial. Ann Intern Med 2016 Jul 19;165(2):77-86. DOI: https://doi.org/10.7326/M15-2143.
52. Nery RM, Zanini M, de Lima JB, et al. Tai Chi Chuan improves functional capacity after myocardial infarction: A randomized clinical trial. Am Heart J 2015 Jun;169(6):854-60. DOI: https://doi.org/10.1016/j.ahj.2015.01.017.
53. Li F, Harmer P, Fitzgerald K, et al. Tai Chi and postural stability in patients with Parkinson's disease. N Engl J Med 2012 Feb 9;366(6):511-19. DOI: https://doi.org/10.1056/NEJMoa1107911.
54. Xiong X, Wang P, Li X, Zhang Y. Qigong for hypertension: A systematic review. Medicine (Baltimore) 2015 Jan;94(1):e352. DOI: https://doi.org/10.1097/MD.0000000000000352.
55. Bai Z, Guan Z, Fan Y, et al. The effects of qigong for adults with chronic pain: Systematic review and meta-analysis. Am J Chin Med 2015;43(8):1525-39. DOI: https://doi.org/10.1142/S0192415X15500871.
56. Anderson JW, Nunnelley PA. Private prayer associations with depression, anxiety and other health conditions: An analytical review of clinical studies. Postgrad Med 2016 Sep;128(7):635-41. DOI: https://doi.org/10.1080/00325481.2016.1209962.
57. Kaplan A. Jewish meditation: A practical guide. New York, NY: Schocken Books; 1995.
58. Finley, J. Christian meditation: Experiencing the presence of god. San Francisco, CA: HarperSanFrancisco; 2004.
59. Kugle S, editor; Ernst C, translator. Sufi meditation and contemplation: Timeless wisdom from Mughal India. New Lebanon, NY: Omega Publications; 2012.
60. Warber SL, DeHudy AA, Bialko MF, Marselle MR, Irvine KN. Addressing "nature-deficit disorder": A mixed methods pilot study of young adults attending a wilderness camp. Evid Based Complement Alternat Med 2015;2015;651827. DOI: https://doi.org/10.1155/2015/651827.

61. Nidich S, Nidich RJ, Salerno J, Hadfield B, Elder C. Stress reduction with the Transcendental Meditation program in caregivers: A pilot study. International Archives of Nursing and Health Care 2015 Nov;1(1):011. DOI: https://doi.org/10.23937/2469-5823/1510011.
62. Desborough MJR, Keeling DM. The aspirin story—from willow to wonder drug. Br J Haematol 2017 Jun;177(5):674-83. DOI: https://doi.org/ 10.1111/bjh.14520.
63. Barrett B, Brown R, Rakel D, et al. Echinacea for treating the common cold: A randomized trial. Ann Intern Med 2010 Dec 21;153(12):769-77. DOI: https://doi.org/10.7326/0003-4819-153-12-201012210-00003.
64. Elder C, Mossbrucker P, Davino-Ramaya CM, et al. Integrating herbs and supplements in managed care: A pharmacy perspective. Perm J 2008 Summer;12(3):52-8. DOI: https://doi.org/10.7812/TPP/07-146.
65. Murphy JJ, Heptinstall S, Mitchell JR. Randomised double-blind placebo-controlled trial of feverfew in migraine prevention. Lancet 1988 Jul 23;2(8604):189-92. DOI: https://doi.org/10.1016/s0140-6736(88)92289-1.
66. Linde K, Berner MM, Kriston L. St John's wort for major depression. Cochrane Database Syst Rev 2008 Oct 8;(4):CD000448. DOI: https://doi.org/10.1002/14651858.CD000448.pub3.
67. Madhu K, Chanda K, Saji MJ. Safety and efficacy of Curcuma longa extract in the treatment of painful knee osteoarthritis: A randomized placebo-controlled trial. Inflammopharmacology 2013 Apr;21(2):129-36. DOI: https://doi.org/10.1007/s10787-012-0163-3.
68. Ziegler D, Ametov A, Barinov A, et al. Oral treatment with alpha-lipoic acid improves symptomatic diabetic polyneuropathy: The SYDNEY 2 trial. Diabetes Care 2006 Nov;29(11):2365-70. DOI: https://doi.org/10.2337/dc06-1216.
69. Caso G, Kelly P, McNurlan MA, Lawson WE. Effect of coenzyme q10 on myopathic symptoms in patients treated with statins. Am J Cardiol 2007 May 15;99(10):1409-12. DOI:10.1016/j.amjcard.2006.12.063.
70. Ferracioli-Oda E, Qawasmi A, Bloch MH. Meta-analysis: Melatonin for the treatment of primary sleep disorders. PLoS One 2013 May 17;8(5):e63773. DOI: https://doi.org/10.1371/journal.pone.0063773.
71. Wu D, Huang Y, Gu Y, Fan W. Efficacies of different preparations of glucosamine for the treatment of osteoarthritis: A meta-analysis of randomised, double-blind, placebo-controlled trials. Int J Clin Pract 2013 Jun;67(6):585-94. DOI: https://doi.org/10.1111/ijcp.12115.
72. Daviglus ML, Stamler J, Orencia AJ, et al. Fish consumption and the 30-year risk of fatal myocardial infarction. N Engl J Med 1997 Apr 10;336(15):1046-53. DOI: https://doi.org/10.1056/NEJM199704103361502.
73. de Roos NM, Katan MB. Effects of probiotic bacteria on diarrhea, lipid metabolism, and carcinogenesis: A review of papers published between 1988 and 1998. Am J Clin Nutr 2000 Feb;71(2):405-11. DOI: https://doi.org/10.1093/ajcn/71.2.405.
74. Hempel S, Newberry SJ, Maher AR, et al. Probiotics for the prevention and treatment of antibiotic-associated diarrhea: A systematic review and meta-analysis. JAMA 2012 May 9;307(18):1959-69. DOI: https://doi.org/10.1001/jama.2012.3507.
75. Halpern GM, Prindiville T, Blankenburg M, Hsia T, Gershwin ME. Treatment of irritable bowel syndrome with Lacteol Fort: A randomized, double-blind, cross-over trial. Am J Gastroenterol 1996 Aug;91(8):1579-85.
76. Science M, Johnstone J, Roth DE, Guyatt G, Loeb M. Zinc for the treatment of the common cold: A systematic review and meta-analysis of randomized controlled trials. CMAJ 2012 Jul 10;184(10):E551-61. DOI: https://doi.org/10.1503/cmaj.111990.
77. Luís Â, Domingues F, Pereira L. Can cranberries contribute to reduce the incidence of urinary tract infections? A systematic review with meta-analysis and trial sequential analysis of clinical trials. J Urol 2017 Sep;198(3):614-21. DOI: https://doi.org/10.1016/j.juro.2017.03.078.
78. Grigoleit HG, Grigoleit P. Peppermint oil in irritable bowel syndrome. Phytomedicine 2005 Aug;12(8):601-6. DOI: https://doi.org/10.1016/j.phymed.2004.10.005.
79. Sengupta K, Alluri KV, Satish AR, et al. A double blind, randomized, placebo controlled study of the efficacy and safety of 5-Loxin for treatment of osteoarthritis of the knee. Arthritis Res Ther 2008;10(4):R85. DOI: https://doi.org/10.1186/ar2461.
80. Morgan A, Stevens J. Does Bacopa monnieri improve memory performance in older persons? Results of a randomized, placebo-controlled, double-blind trial. J Altern Complement Med 2010 Jul;16(7):753-9. DOI: https://doi.org/ 10.1089/acm.2009.0342.
81. Chandrasekhar K, Kapoor J, Anishetty S. A prospective, randomized double-blind, placebo-controlled study of safety and efficacy of a high-concentration full-spectrum extract of ashwagandha root in reducing stress and anxiety in adults. Indian J Psychol Med 2012 Jul;34(3):255-62. DOI: https://doi.org/10.4103/0253-7176.106022.

82. Ritenbaugh C, Hammershlag R, Dworkin SF, et al. Comparative effectiveness of traditional Chinese medicine and psychosocial care in the treatment of temporomandibular disorders-associated chronic facial pain. J Pain 2012 Nov;13(11):1075-98. DOI: https://doi.org/10.1016/j.jpain.2012.08.002.
83. Fortmann SP, Burda BU, Senger CA, Lin JS, Whitlock EP. Vitamin and mineral supplements in the primary prevention of cardiovascular disease and cancer: An updated systematic evidence review for the US Preventive Services Task Force. Ann Intern Med 2013 Dec 17;159(12):824-34. DOI: https://doi.org/10.7326/0003-4819-159-12-201312170-00729.
84. Merriam-Webster [Internet]. Springfield (MA): Merriam-Webster, Incorporated; c2019. Available from: www.merriam-webster.com.
85. Kaptchuk TJ, Kelley JM, Conboy LA, et al. Components of placebo effect: Randomised controlled trial in patients with irritable bowel syndrome. BMJ 2008 May 3;336(7651):999-1003. DOI: https://doi.org/ 10.1136/bmj.39524.439618.25.
86. Cherkin DC, Sherman KJ, Avins AL, et al. A randomized trial comparing acupuncture, simulated acupuncture, and usual care for chronic low back pain. Arch Intern Med 2009 May 11;169(9):858-66. DOI: https://doi.org/ 10.1001/archinternmed.2009.65.
87. Vickers AJ, Cronin AM, Maschino AC, et al; Acupuncture Trialists' Collaboration. Acupuncture for chronic pain: Individual patient data meta-analysis. Arch Intern Med 2012 Oct 22;172(19):1444-53. DOI: https://doi.org/10.1001/archinternmed.2012.3654.
88. Bronfort G, Haas M, Evans R, Leininger B, Triano J. Effectiveness of manual therapies: The UK evidence report. Chiropr Osteopat 2010 Feb 25;18:3. DOI: https://doi.org/10.1186/1746-1340-18-3.
89. Furlan AD, Imamura M, Dryden T, Irvin E. Massage for l ow-back pain. Cochrane Database Syst Rev 2008 Oct;8(4):CD001929. DOI: https://doi.org/ 10.1002/14651858.CD001929.pub2.
90. Penney LS, Ritenbaugh C, DeBar LL, Elder C, Deyo RA. Provider and patient perspectives on opioids and alternative treatments for managing chronic pain: A qualitative study. BMC Fam Pract 2017 Mar 24;17(1):164. DOI: https://doi.org/10.1186/s12875-016-0566-0.
91. House of Delegates position paper: Definition of naturopathic medicine [Internet]. Washington, DC: American Association of Naturopathic Physicians; 1989 [amended 2011; cited 2017 Jun 20]. Available from: www.naturopathic.org/files/Committees/HOD/Position%20Paper%20Docs/Definition%20Naturopathic%20Medicine.pdf.
92. Elder CR. Integrating naturopathy: Can we move forward? Perm J 2013 Fall;17(4):80-3. DOI: https://doi.org/10.7812/TPP/13-034.
93. Ritenbaugh C, Verhoef M, Fleishman S, Boon H, Leis A. Whole systems research: A discipline for studying complementary and alternative medicine. Altern Ther Health Med 2003 Jul-Aug;9(4):32-6.
94. Ritenbaugh C, Hammerschlag R, Calabrese C, et al. A pilot whole systems clinical trial of traditional Chinese medicine and naturopathic medicine for the treatment of temporomandibular disorders. J Altern Complement Med 2008 Jun;14(5):475-87. DOI: https://doi.org/10.1089/acm.2007.0738.
95. Grozlnsky-Glasberg S, Fraser A, Nahshoni E, Weizman A, Leibovici L. Thyroxine-triiodothyronine combination therapy versus thyroxine monotherapy for clinical hypothyroidism: Meta-analysis of randomized controlled trials. J Clin Endocrinol Metab 2006 Jul;91(7):2592-9. DOI: https://doi.org/10.1210/jc.2006-0448.
96. Hamre HJ, Kiene H, Kienle GS. Clinical research in anthroposophic medicine. Altern Ther Health Med 2009 Nov-Dec;15(6):52-5.
97. Linde K, Melchart D. Randomized controlled trials of individualized homeopathy: A state-of-the-art review. J Altern Complement Med 1998 Winter;4(4):371-88. DOI: https://doi.org/10.1089/acm.1998.4.371.
98. Functional medicine [Internet]. Federal Way, WA: The Institute for Functional Medicine; 2018 [cited 2017 Jun 20]. Available from: www.functionalmedicine.org/What_is_Functional_Medicine/AboutFM.
99. Chen L, Michalsen A. Management of chronic pain using complementary and integrative medicine. BMJ 2017 Apr 24;357:j1284. DOI: https://doi.org/ https://doi.org/10.1136/bmj.j1284.
100. Müller H, de Toledo FW, Resch KL. Fasting followed by vegetarian diet in patients with rheumatoid arthritis: A systematic review. Scand J Rheumatol 2001;30(1):1-10. DOI: https://doi.org/10.1080/030097401750065256.

101. Herron RE, Fagan JB. Lipophil-mediated reduction of toxicants in humans: An evaluation of an ayurvedic detoxification procedure. Altern Ther Health Med 2002 Sep-Oct;8(5):40-51.
102. Sharma HM, Nidich SI, Sands D, Smith DE. Improvements in cardiovascular risk factors through Panchakarma purification procedures. J Res Educ Indian Med 1993;12(4):3-13.
103. Bertozzi L, Gardenghi I, Turoni F, et al. Effect of therapeutic exercise on pain and disability in the management of chronic nonspecific neck pain: Systematic review and meta-analysis of randomized trials. Phys Ther 2013 Aug;93(8):1026-36. DOI: https://doi.org/10.2522/ptj.20120412.
104. Gill SD, McBurney H. Does exercise reduce pain and improve physical function before hip or knee replacement surgery? A systematic review and meta-analysis of randomized controlled trials. Arch Phys Med Rehabil 2013 Jan;94(1):164-76. DOI: https://doi.org/10.1016/j.apmr.2012.08.211.
105. Smith DE, Salerno JW. Selective growth inhibition of a human malignant melanoma cell line by sesame oil in vitro. Prostaglandins Leukot Essent Fatty Acids 1992 Jun;46(2):145-50. DOI: https://doi.org/10.1016/0952-3278(92)90221-4.
106. Fukuda Y, Nagata M, Osawa T, Namiki M. Contribution of lignin analogues to antioxidative activity of refined unroasted sesame oil. Journal of the American Oil Chemists' Society 1986 Aug;63(8):1027-31. DOI: https://doi.org/10.1007/bf02673792.
107. Monteiro EM, Chibli LA, Yamamoto CH, et al. Antinociceptive and anti-inflammatory activities of the sesame oil and sesamin. Nutrients 2014 May 12;6(5):1931-44. DOI: https://doi.org/10.3390/nu6051931.
108. Bigdeli Shamloo MB, Nasiri M, Dabirian A, Bakhtiyari A, Mojab F, Alavi Majd H. The effects of topical sesame (Sesamum indicum) oil on pain severity and amount of received non-steroid anti-inflammatory drugs in patients with upper or lower extremities trauma. Anesth Pain Med 2015 Jun 22;5(3):e25085. DOI: https://doi.org/10.5812/aapm.25085v2.
109. Asokan S, Emmadi P, Chamundeswari R. Effect of oil pulling on plaque induced gingivitis: A randomized, controlled, triple-blind study. Indian J Dent Res 2009 Jan-Mar;20(1):47-51. DOI: https://doi.org/10.4103/0970-9290.49067.
110. Gbinigie O, Onakpoya I, Spencer E, McCall MacBain M, Heneghan C. Effect of oil pulling in promoting oro dental hygiene: A systematic review of randomized clinical trials. Complement Ther Med 2016 Jun;26:47-54. DOI: https://doi.org/ 10.1016/j.ctim.2016.02.011.
111. MacPherson H, Tilbrook H, Richmond S, et al. Alexander technique lessons or acupuncture sessions for persons with chronic neck pain: A randomized trial. Ann Intern Med 2015 Nov 3;163(9):653-62. DOI: https://doi.org/10.1186/1745-6215-14-209.
112. Lundqvist LO, Zetterlund C, Richter HO. Effects of Feldenkrais method on chronic neck/scapular pain in people with visual impairment: A randomized controlled trial with one-year follow-up. Arch Phys Med Rehabil 2014 Sep;95(9):1656-61. DOI: https://doi.org/10.1016/j.apmr.2014.05.013.
113. Karaman T, Karaman S, Dogru S, et al. Evaluating the efficacy of lavender aromatherapy on peripheral venous cannulation pain and anxiety: A prospective, randomized study. Complement Ther Clin Pract 2016 May;23:64-8. DOI: https://doi.org/10.1016/j.ctcp.2016.03.008.
114. Elder C. Ayurveda for diabetes mellitus: A review of the biomedical literature. Altern Ther Health Med 2004 Jan-Feb;10(1):44-50.
115. Paul-Labrador M, Polk D, Dwyer JH, et al. Effects of a randomized controlled trial of transcendental meditation on components of the metabolic syndrome in subjects with coronary heart disease. Arch Intern Med 2006 Jun 12;166(11):1218-24. DOI: https://doi.org/10.1001/archinte.166.11.1218.
116. Younge JO, Leening MJ, Tiemeier H, et al. Association between mind-body practice and cardiometabolic risk factors: The Rotterdam Study. Psychosom Med 2015 Sep;77(7):775-83. DOI: https://doi.org/10.1097/PSY.0000000000000213.
117. Allen RW, Schwartzman E, Baker WL, Coleman CI, Phung OJ. Cinnamon use in type 2 diabetes: An updated systematic review and meta-analysis. Ann Fam Med 2013 Sep-Oct;11(5):452-9. DOI: https://doi.org/10.1370/afm.1517.
118. Neelakantan N, Narayanan M, de Souza RJ, van Dam RM. Effect of fenugreek (Trigonella foenum-graecum L.) intake on glycemia: A meta-analysis of clinical trials. Nutr J 2014 Jan 18;13:7. DOI: https://doi.org/10.1186/1475-2891-13-7.

119. Balk EM, Tatsioni A, Lichtenstein AH, Lau J, Pittas AG. Effect of chromium supplementation on glucose metabolism and lipids: A systematic review of randomized controlled trials. Diabetes Care 2007 Aug;30(8):2154-63. DOI: https://doi.org/10.2337/dc06-0996.
120. Lee Y, Park K. Adherence to a vegetarian diet and diabetes risk: A systematic review and meta-analysis of observational studies. Nutrients 2017 Jun 14;9(6):603. DOI: https://doi.org/10.3390/nu9060603.
121. Pawlak R. Vegetarian diets in the prevention and management of diabetes and its complications. Diabetes Spectr 2017 May;30(2):82-8. DOI: https://doi.org/10.2337/ds16-0057.
122. Castillo-Richmond A, Schneider RH, Alexander CN, et al. Effects of stress reduction on carotid atherosclerosis in hypertensive African Americans. Stroke 2000 Mar;31(3):568-73. DOI: https://doi.org/10.1161/01.str.31.3.568.
123. Zamarra JW, Schneider RH, Besseghini I, Robinson DK, Salerno JW. Usefulness of the transcendental meditation program in the treatment of patients with coronary artery disease. Am J Cardiol 1996 Apr 15;77(10):867-70. DOI: https://doi.org/10.1016/s0002-9149(97)89184-9.
124. Acosta-Navarro J, Antoniazzi L, Oki AM, et al. Reduced subclinical carotid vascular disease and arterial stiffness in vegetarian men: The CARVOS Study. Int J Cardiol 2017 Mar 1;230:562-6. DOI: https://doi.org/ 10.1016/j.ijcard.2016.12.058.
125. Liu J, Zhang J, Shi Y, Grimsgaard S, Alraek T, Fønnebø V. Chinese red yeast rice (Monascus purpureus) for primary hyperlipidemia: A meta-analysis of randomized controlled trials. Chin Med 2006 Nov 23;1:4. DOI: https://doi.org/10.1186/1749-8546-1-4.
126. Nityanand S, Srivastava JS, Asthana OP. Clinical trials with gugulipid. A new hypolipidaemic agent. J Assoc Physicians India 1989 May;37(5):323-8.
127. Szapary PO, Wolfe ML, Bloedon LT, et al. Guggulipid for treatment of hypercholesterolemia: A randomized controlled trial. JAMA 2003 Aug 13;290(6):765-72. DOI: https://doi.org/10.1001/jama.290.6.765.
128. Sugiyama T, Tsugawa Y, Tseng CH, Kabayashi Y, Shapiro MF. Different time trends of caloric and fat intake between statin users and nonusers among US adults: Gluttony in the time of statins? JAMA Intern Med 2014 Jul;174(7):1038-45. DOI: https://doi.org/10.1001/jamainternmed.2014.1927.
129. Nidich SI, Fields JZ, Rainforth MV, et al. A randomized controlled trial of the effects of transcendental meditation on quality of life in older breast cancer patients. Integr Cancer Ther 2009 Sep;8(3):228-34. DOI: https://doi.org/10.1177/1534735409343000.
130. Vickers AJ. Can acupuncture have specific effects on health? A systematic review of acupuncture antiemesis trials. J R Soc Med 1996 Jun;89(6):303-11. DOI: https://doi.org/10.1177/014107689608900602.
131. Fraser GE. Vegetarian diets: What do we know of their effects on common chronic diseases? Am J Clin Nutr 2009 May;89(5):1607S-12S. DOI: https://doi.org/ 10.3945/ajcn.2009.26736K.
132. Penza M, Montani C, Jeremic M, et al. MAK-4 and -5 supplemented diet inhibits liver carcinogenesis in mice. BMC Complement Altern Med 2007 Jun 8;7:19. DOI: https://doi.org/10.1186/1472-6882-7-19.
133. Prasad ML, Parry P, Chan C. Ayurvedic agents produce differential effects on murine and human melanoma cells in vitro. Nutr Cancer 1993;20(1):79-86. DOI: https://doi.org/10.1080/01635589309514273.
134. Vohra BP, Sharma SP, Kansal VK. Maharishi Amrit Kalash rejuvenates ageing central nervous system's antioxidant defence system: An in vivo study. Pharmacol Res 1999 Dec;40(6):497-502. DOI: https://doi.org/10.1006/phrs.1999.0540.
135. Vohra BP, Sharma SP, Kansal VK. Effect of Maharishi Amrit Kalash on age dependent variations in mitochondrial antioxidant enzymes, lipid peroxidation and mitochondrial population in different regions of the central nervous system of guinea-pigs. Drug Metabol Drug Interact 2001;18(1):57-68. DOI: https://doi.org/10.1515/dmdi.2001.18.1.57.
136. Dwivedi C, Agrawal P, Natarajan K, Sharma H. Antioxidant and protective effects of Amrit Nectar tablets on adriamycin- and cisplatin-induced toxicities. J Altern Complement Med 2005 Feb;11(1):143-8. DOI: https://doi.org/10.1089/acm.2005.11.143.
137. Dich J, Zahm SH, Hanberg A, Adami HO. Pesticides and cancer. Cancer Causes Control 1997 May;8(3):420-43. DOI: https://doi.org/10.1023/A:1018413522959.
138. Sood R, Warndahl RA, Schroeder DR, et al. Bioidentical compounded hormones: A pharmacokinetic evaluation in a randomized clinical trial. Maturitas 2013 Apr;74(4):375-82. DOI: https://doi.org/10.1016/j.maturitas.2013.01.010.

139. Shams T, Setia MS, Hemmings R, McCusker J, Sewitch M, Ciampi A. Efficacy of black cohosh-containing preparations on menopausal symptoms: A meta-analysis. Altern Ther Health Med 2010 Jan-Feb;16(1):36-44.
140. Del-Pino-Casado R, Obrero-Gaitán E, Lomas-Vega R. The effect of tai chi on reducing the risk of falling: A systematic review and meta-analysis. Am J Chin Med 2016;44(5):895-906. DOI: https://doi.org/ 10.1142/S0192415X1650049X.
141. Bilezikian JP. Efficacy of bisphosphonates in reducing fracture risk in postmenopausal osteoporosis. Am J Med 2009 Feb;122(2 Suppl):S14-21. DOI: https://doi.org/10.1016/j.amjmed.2008.12.003.
142. Meunier PJ, Roux C, Seeman E, et al. The effects of strontium ranelate on the risk of vertebral fracture in women with postmenopausal osteoporosis. N Engl J Med 2004 Jan 29;350(5):459-68. DOI: https://doi.org/10.1056/NEJMoa022436.
143. Yang M, Xu DD, Zhang Y, Liu X, Hoeven R, Cho WC. A systematic review on natural medicines for the prevention and treatment of Alzheimer's disease with meta-analyses of intervention effect of ginkgo. Am J Chin Med 2014;42(3):505-21. DOI: https://doi.org/10.1142/S0192415X14500335.
144. Swing EL, Gentile DA, Anderson CA, Walsh DA. Television and video game exposure and the development of attention problems. Pediatrics 2010 Aug;126(2):214-21. DOI: https://doi.org/10.1542/peds.2009-1508.
145. Radesky J, Christakis D; Council on Communications and Media. Media and young minds. Pediatrics 2016 Nov;138(5):e20162591. DOI: https://doi.org/10.1542/peds.2016-2591.
146. Reid Chassiakos Y, Radesky J, Christakis D, Moreno MA, Cross C; Council on Communications and Media. Children and adolescents and digital media. Pediatrics 2016 Nov;138(5):e20162593. DOI: https://doi.org/10.1542/peds.2016-2593.
147. Doshi P, Stahl-Timmins W, Merino JG, Simpkins C. Visualising childhood vaccination schedules across G8 countries. BMJ 2015 Nov 15;351:h5966. DOI: https://doi.org/10.1136/bmj.h5966.
148. Musher D. Pneumococcal vaccination in adults [Internet]. Waltham, MA: UpToDate; 2018 [updated 2018 Feb 27; cited 2017 Jul 30]. Available from: www.uptodate.com/contents/pneumococcal-vaccination-in-adults.

ACKNOWLEDGMENTS

We would like to take a moment to thank the many wonderful friends and colleagues who have contributed to this project. A few individuals warrant special mention. In particular, we wish to express our gratitude to Laura McArdle, who, in addition to being a terrific friend and neighbor, is also a superb photographer who helped us immensely with the reproductions of the artwork. Likewise, our nephew, Noah Elder, is a skilled graphic artist and assisted us in developing the various charts and graphics for the text.

Finally, we are extremely grateful to the staff at The Permanente Press, including Tom Janisse, Merry Parker, Max McMillen, Lynette Leisure, Amy Watson-Terry, Ian Kimmich, and Katy Drawhorn. This outstanding team of professionals have generously offered their time and expertise, and have supported and encouraged us over a period of years to make this book possible.

INDEX

ABOUT THE AUTHORS

Charles R. Elder, MD, MPH, FACP, received his MD and MPH degrees from Boston University School of Medicine, and completed residency training in internal medicine at the University of Michigan hospitals. He has served as a primary care internist at Kaiser Permanente Northwest (KPNW) for 26 years and has been the physician lead for the complementary and integrative medicine program at KPNW for 18 years. In this capacity, Dr. Elder offers a referral-based integrative ayurvedic clinic for KPNW patients, advising patients in the areas of diet, exercise, herbal medicine, mind-body practices, and other complementary medicine modalities. He has also provided leadership in shaping and implementing policy related to management of chiropractic, acupuncture, naturopathy, and other complementary medicine benefits. Dr. Elder holds a Senior Investigator appointment at the Kaiser Permanente Center for Health Research, where he has served as principal or co-investigator on a range of federally funded studies evaluating mind-body and other complementary medicine interventions in the setting of chronic disease management. He also has a clinical faculty appointment at Oregon Health and Science University, and for more than 2 decades has mentored and taught residents and students in both internal and integrative medicine settings. He has published 59 articles and abstracts in peer-reviewed scientific journals, and his research has been widely publicized in local, national, and international media outlets.

Leslie D. Elder, MD, received her MD degree from the University of Nevada School of Medicine, and completed residency training in family medicine at the University of Michigan hospitals. She practiced urgency care medicine for 15 years, during which time she also maintained a private integrative medicine practice focused on ayurvedic herbal and dietary therapeutics. Dr. Elder is both an accomplished gourmet vegetarian cook as well as a talented visual artist (www.leslieelder.com). Her work has been displayed in multiple venues through ORA Northwest Jewish Artists, the Oregon Watercolor Society, and in other settings. She is a member of the Oregon Society of Artists.